WHAT YO[U]
NEED[ TO]
KNO[W]

# THYROID PROBLEMS

## DR TOM SMITH

WELLHOUSE

First published in the United Kingdom in 2001 by

Wellhouse Publishing Ltd
604 The Chandlery
50 Westminster Bridge Road
LONDON
SE1 7QY
Email: info@wellhousepublishing.co.uk

Reprinted in 2003, 2004, 2005, 2006, 2010, 2012.

## DISCLAIMER

The aim of this book is to provide general information only and should not be treated as a substitute for the medical advice of your doctor or any other health care professional. The publisher and author is not responsible or liable for any diagnosis made by a reader based on the contents of this book. Always consult your doctor if you are in any way concerned about your health.

ISBN 978-1-903784-37-2

Printed and bound in the United Kingdom

# Contents

# Introduction

Why a whole book on the thyroid? It's not a subject that immediately springs to mind when we chat socially about our health. Weight problems usually take the first priority. How to cope with being too fat is probably number one, followed closely by being too thin, particularly for women (though, increasingly, men as well) today, under pressure from media images such as those in fashion magazines and television programmes.

Another common obsession is with energy levels. We marvel at the way some people seem to have boundless energy, can eat like a horse and still be as thin as a lath, while others (usually ourselves) are always tired and weary, and overweight even when we eat half as much. We have invented 'TATT' – Tired All The Time syndrome – to describe this state of slowing down, mentally and physically.

Then there are 'nervous' states. We all recognize them. There's the anxious, agitated, hot, sweaty person who can never sit still. It's only too easy to label such people as suffering from a continual 'anxiety state'. And then there's the tired, couldn't care less, miserable people whose main interest revolves around how to manage constipation. They are presumed, of course, to be 'depressed', and treated accordingly, often with little sympathy or understanding.

It is all too easy to assume that people differ in these ways because of their characters or their lifestyles. Then *they* can be blamed for their problems, and be told that they must change the way they live. That is an easy way out for relatives and health professionals, who then don't have to get to grips with the true underlying causes of the symptoms.

## The Role of the Thyroid Gland in Our Health

It is true that many people who are too fat eat too much and exercise too little, and that many people who are too thin are overactive and over-anxious. Such people do have to re-organize their lives. But a substantial minority have become the way they have through no fault of their own. Their body's 'accelerator pedal' – the thyroid gland – has gone wrong. It may always be pressed down to the boards, in which case no matter how hard they try these people will burn up fuel far too fast. Or the accelerator pedal may not be working at all, and the body remains sluggish and operates only at the slowest speed.

Working just right, the thyroid gland helps to keep us in normal physical and mental shape. When it goes wrong it affects our every action, our thinking, our mood and even our ability to reason. It is small wonder that thyroid disease can mimic so many other illnesses, and that it often escapes notice, even by the professionals.

## Underactive Thyroid

Take, for example, the woman complaining of tiredness, apathy, constipation and depression. All these symptoms have come on fairly recently, and her partner states that she is quite different from her normal, cheerful self. Her doctor, instead of jumping to the conclusion that she has depression, examines her thyroid gland with gentle fingers. It is slightly swollen, firm, a little knobbly, but not tender. The likely cause is not a psychiatric illness, but an underactive thyroid (hypothyroidism). A condition called Hashimoto's thyroiditis (see Chapter Four) affects the hormone output from the thyroid, making it lower than normal. Once blood tests have confirmed this diagnosis, treatment is an almost instantaneous success: within hours she will be feeling better, and within days she will be back to her previous self.

## Overactive Thyroid

The other side of the thyroid coin is the woman who is ravenously hungry and eats accordingly. Yet she is losing weight. Shaking hands with her you feel a warm, wet palm. Watch her reading a paper, and you see it tremble in her hands. She may complain of palpitations – a fluttering feeling in her chest – and she feels weaker than she used to, particularly after only slight exertion. Her eyes may have become more prominent than before. Her thyroid, to the doctor's touch, feels smoothly swollen.

This is classically the person with an overactive thyroid (hyperthyroidism), where there's a higher than normal thyroid hormone output – her accelerator pedal is down to the floor and she is speeding out of control. Again, it only needs simple blood tests to confirm the condition. Her treatment, however, is a bit more complex than that for the underactive gland.

These are the two classical thyroid problems, and if you have picked up this book because you, or someone close to you, have a thyroid problem, it's more than likely that you recognize one or other of these two pictures. But they are by no means the complete picture of how thyroid disease may present itself.

## OtherThyroid Problems

Take people who come to the doctor with a fever and sore throat. Of course, in most cases these symptoms are caused by an infection in the throat and tonsils, and need treatment accordingly. But doctors in training are always taught, as a routine, to feel the patient's thyroid glands. Because if they don't, they will miss the occasional person whose thyroid is exquisitely tender. This is a condition called 'subacute thyroiditis': it can lead to later complications and needs thorough investigation.

Then there is the person who has become short of breath over the past few months. It is so easy, without bothering to examine the thyroid, to make the diagnosis of asthma or chronic bronchitis. But a suspicion of an enlarged thyroid gland low in the throat may mean that there is a much larger portion of it lying behind the upper part of the breastbone. Because it is jammed into a confined space, it compresses the windpipe (trachea). This is what has caused the breathlessness – in effect strangling the person from the inside. Obviously this is a problem that cannot be overlooked.

Some people have noticed their thyroid trouble themselves. They come to the doctor because their necks are lumpy – they have a 'goitre'. Most such thyroid lumps are quite harmless, and leave the 'accelerator' in neutral, so that the people who possess them feel and are their normal selves. But these problems should be looked at professionally, because they can cause trouble.

For example, there is the person who has a small thyroid lump and a hoarse voice. This may indicate that the nerve to the voice-box (larynx) has been affected by the lump – and this can be a sign of thyroid cancer. Thyroid cancer is very rare, so if you have a goitre, don't jump to the wrong conclusions. But it must be ruled out with any abnormal thyroid swelling, so don't hesitate in getting help once you have found one.

People already being treated with thyroid hormone (thyroxine is the most usual) should also be mentioned here. They belong to one of two general groups. The most obvious are people who need thyroid hormone treatment because their thyroid has stopped working – this is again called hypothyroidism, or sometimes myxoedema. The second group comprises people who used to have an overactive thyroid, but whose treatment has left them with lower than normal thyroid activity, and who therefore need the extra thyroid hormone in pill form.

In either case, once they have started on thyroxine treatment, the thyroid gland shrinks away virtually to nothing, so that the doctor can no longer feel it. If it can still be felt in such circumstances, then something is not right – either its structure is abnormal, or it is working away on its own, without reacting to the body's normal control systems. That, too, needs investigating.

Besides the usual thyroid problems in the average adult, thyroid disease can also affect newborn babies, older children, and pregnant and nursing women. They all pose their special problems. So the question that opens this book has been answered: thyroid problems do merit a whole book.

## About This Book

The pages that follow explain where the thyroid gland is, what it does, how the body's control systems keep it in check, the various ways in which it can go wrong, and how they show up in symptoms and illness. It takes you through the tests and treatments for the common, and some less common, thyroid diseases. It is meant for the lay person with no special medical knowledge, who may be interested because they or a partner or relative have thyroid trouble, and who want to know more than their medical team has time to explain.

## How Thyroid Disease Affects the Rest of the Body

Although I have described the thyroid as our accelerator – the organ that determines the speed with which all our body's functions work – it is much more than that. When it goes wrong, all sorts of organs suffer. The heart speeds up or slows down, depending on whether the thyroid is over- or underactive, but its rhythm can also go awry. And that can be more significant than the rate change. The skin changes, too, in both forms of thyroid disease. The muscles and nerves may not work at their best, leaving people weaker than expected. The brain can slow down and moods can change. The bowel, again depending on the hormone output, can be over- or underactive, leading to diarrhoea or constipation.

In effect, therefore, thyroid trouble can mimic many other illnesses, and the symptoms can sometimes lead the doctor down a wrong diagnostic track before their true significance becomes apparent. Any doctor can tell embarrassing tales of mistaken diagnoses made of dementia, depression, anxiety neurosis, heart disease and muscular and nervous disorders until the penny dropped and the thyroid disease was confirmed. This book will cover that ground, too, and hopefully will help in a small way to prevent such mistakes. It is vital that it does, because most thyroid disease is eminently treatable, and the treatment almost always restores people to a normal life and life expectancy. That is more than can be said of many of the conditions with which it can be confused.

Mistakes can be made in the other direction. At the 2000 conference of the British Endocrine Societies, alarming news was given about people who were suffering unnecessary illness because they were taking thyroxine when their thyroid glands were in fact normal. The paper that caused most concern was from Dr Peter Daggett, of Stafford, and Dr Terry West, of Telford, who reported on patients whose thyroxine treatment had been started purely on the basis of their symptoms, without blood tests having been done. When these patients were eventually investigated, their thyroids were found to be normal.

One of these patients, who had been previously healthy, had been put into heart failure by her unnecessary thyroxine treatment. Dr Daggett reported:

Some doctors do not believe the thyroid function tests and are giving thyroxine to people with normal function. This can cause problems to their circulation and their bones. I am now seeing about one patient a month in Stafford. They are usually middle-aged ladies who complain of feeling run down. The treatment may well make you feel much better in the short-term, but it is as if they have become addicted to the treatment.

At the same meeting, Dr Anne Pollock, of Glasgow, described the flood of people who diagnosed themselves as hypothyroid (with lowered thyroid activity) after a series of articles in local newspapers on the subject. Many were given the thyroid hormone thyroxine purely on the basis that they had symptoms suggestive of thyroid disease. Dr Pollock described 25 people who were taking thyroxine despite tests showing that their thyroid glands were normal. She and her colleagues found that thyroxine was no better than placebo at making them feel better, and did not improve their health.

So the last thing in my mind as I write this book is to encourage people to take thyroid hormones if they do not need to do so. This book is for people who have thyroid disease and their friends and families. It is not to promote the use of self-treatment for and self-diagnosis of thyroid problems. Never take thyroxine unless there is a good medical reason for it. It should never be used as a 'pick-me-up', or, in particular, as a way to lose weight. That, too, has been an abuse of thyroxine for many years.

One last point. Far more women than men develop thyroid problems. For grammatical convenience I have therefore used 'she' and 'her' when writing about people with these problems. For the most part, though, what I have written about thyroid disease is applicable equally to both sexes. Where it is not, this is mentioned in the text.

# Part One
# The Thyroid – How It Works

# Chapter One

# The Normal Thyroid

## Where it is:

The thyroid gland lies just below and to the sides of the Adam's apple (larynx), in front of the windpipe (trachea), in the U-shaped notch formed by the top of the breastbone (sternum) and the inner ends of the collarbones (see diagram). It is best seen, if it can be seen at all, if the person tilts her head backwards. That raises it up from behind the sternum and throws the swelling of the gland into relief against the underlying neck structures. If the person swallows a small amount of water in this position, the thyroid can be seen moving first upwards, then down again.

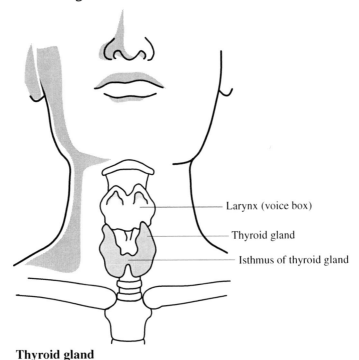

Larynx (voice box)

Thyroid gland

Isthmus of thyroid gland

**Thyroid gland**

Observing a normal thyroid needs practice, and in people with fairly fat necks this can be particularly difficult. In fact, some medical text-books state that the normal thyroid gland cannot usually be seen or felt. Other textbook authors say that they find it relatively easy. My experience as a general practitioner suggests to me that it probably takes a thyroid specialist's expertise to feel a normal thyroid. On the other hand, if the gland is enlarged or contains a lump, then it is plain to the untrained eye and its abnormal 'feel' is obvious to doctors like myself.

Excess fat in the neck does not rise and fall when we swallow, unlike the thyroid gland which is attached to the trachea. This is one way to tell the difference between a 'goitre' – an enlarged thyroid – and a horizontal band of fat in the neck. The thyroid rises and falls; the fat remains at the same level. It is an important distinction, as fatty necks are much more common than thyroid swellings and of course need quite a different medical approach.

The normal thyroid is wrapped around the front of the top of the tra-chea, just below the cricoid, the lowest cartilage of the larynx. It has a dumbbell shape, with a wing or 'lobe' on either side, and a bar or 'isth-mus' joining the two (see diagram). In a person with a thin neck the isthmus can sometimes be felt if the thumb is placed on the midline of the neck just underneath the larynx as the person swallows. It is about a centimetre in width (from above down) and about two centi-metres long (horizontally). In older men, especially if they have chronic bronchitis and 'hunch' their necks into their chests, the cri-coid cartilage lies lower in the neck, and it is virtually impossible to feel the isthmus, or in fact the lobes. Such men often need a barium X-ray to detect the site and size of their thyroid.

Doctors like myself were trained to feel the thyroid from behind the patient, with her seated in a chair and the chin tilted slightly down-wards, so that the large neck muscles from the sternum to the back of the ear – the sternomastoids – are loose and relaxed. We then feel for the thyroid lobes with the fingertips of both hands. We were taught that this was the best way to judge the texture (smoothness) and size of the gland.

Today's medical students are offered the choice of this method or feeling for the thyroid from the front. To do this, the doctor stands to the patient's right, and places the index and middle fingers of the right hand against the side of her trachea, so that they lie in the fold between the sternomastoid muscle and the centre of the throat. The fingers are then drawn down the side of the trachea, massaging it with constant pressure as they go, while the patient takes sips of water. This gives the doctor a good idea of the health or otherwise of the left thyroid lobe: it shows whether the lobe is of the right size, consistency and smoothness, or whether it is enlarged, shrunken, too hard, lumpy or tender. The doctor then repeats the examination standing on the patient's left side, using the left hand in the same manner.

The examination may end with the doctor listening to the thyroid with a stethoscope. In some people with a swollen thyroid and symptoms of overactivity, the stethoscope can pick up a continuous low-pitched hum (a 'venous hum') or a murmur linked to the heartbeat (a 'bruit'). These suggest that the blood flow through the gland is much greater than normal and that the gland's hormone output is accordingly much higher. These observations tend to confirm the diagnosis of an overactive thyroid (hyperthyroidism or thyrotoxicosis).

## What It Does – The Role of Thyroxine

The thyroid is an endocrine gland. This means that it produces within it a substance – a hormone – which is secreted directly into the bloodstream and which has profound effects on distant organs. In the thyroid's case the main hormone is thyroxine, although it also produces two others, tri-iodothyronine and calcitonin. The following paragraphs explain what these hormones do, but it's also important to know a little about the basic 'building bricks' of these hormones, because they help us to understand why some people develop thyroid problems and how they can be solved and cured.

Here, a little history of the medical research into the thyroid may be appropriate. The ancient Greeks and Romans recognized swellings in the throat which were obviously what we now know of as enlarged thyroid glands. The Roman physicians Pliny and Juvenal used the term *tumid guttur* – swollen throat – which has come down to us in the word *goitre*, universally known now as a thyroid disease.

Not that these respected doctors knew much about what the thyroid did. In 1711 the Italian professor J Vercelloni was writing that the thyroid was a bag of worms, the eggs of which crossed for digestive purposes into the oesophagus (the gullet). How exactly this helped digestion was not explained. The real breakthrough in understanding the thyroid came in 1883, when two different groups of surgeons in Germany (led by T Kocher) and Switzerland (J L and A Reverdin) reported on what happened to patients whose goitres they had removed surgically. A huge academic row ensued over who had been first to recognize that the illness myxoedema (extreme hypothyroidism, or underactivity of the thyroid) and the illness that followed the removal of goitres were the same.

The direct connection between myxoedema and lack of thyroid activity was finally made in 1891, when the British doctor G R Murray reported on the cure of myxoedema by injections of a glycerine extract of sheep thyroid glands into his patients. He was fortunate: none of his patients seems to have reacted badly to the injection of such 'foreign' proteins. We would not dare copy his method today for fear of inducing a fatal allergic reaction. Much safer and just as effective was the feeding of lightly cooked sheep thyroid glands to patients with an underactive thyroid, as undertaken by Dr F Vermeulen in 1893.

From then on it was only a matter of time before the real active ingredient in thyroid glands was identified chemically and could be used as a pure substance. By 1915 pure thyroxine had been crystallized (by the American E C Kendall) and by 1927 C R Harington and G Barger, in the United Kingdom, had published its detailed chemical structure. From then on patients with an underactive thyroid could be given a pure thyroid hormone in an exact dose which could be altered precisely to suit each one of them.

This thyroid hormone, thyroxine, is still the mainstay of the management of many thyroid disorders today. It is taken daily by people who have been treated for an overactive thyroid, to regulate their hormone levels, and by people with myxoedema.

At its simplest, the symptoms of an overactive thyroid are caused by an excess of thyroxine in the circulation, and the symptoms of an underactive thyroid are caused by its low levels or complete absence. To understand why these symptoms arise, we have to understand what thyroxine actually does in people with normal thyroid glands.

First of all, thyroxine affects every tissue, in that it controls the speed at which each cell conducts its 'business'. With normal levels of thyroid hormone, everything ticks along normally. So the fat cells release just enough fat when asked to do so; the muscle cells, including those in the heart, contract at the right speed and tension; the

16

brain cells pass on their messages at the normal rate and in the usual number; the liver cells control the amount of glucose released to the bloodstream at the usual rate, and so on.

Too much thyroxine leads to all these processes speeding up even when the body is at rest, so that the heart beats faster even during sleep, and the muscles tremble and become weak and waste away, because of the constant extra demand on them. The fat in our energy storage cells becomes used up, and even the most prodigious appetite cannot stop people losing weight. The brain becomes overactive, and with that can come anxiety and agitation.

With low thyroxine output, the reverse of these symptoms occur. The heart, brain and other tissues slow down. The heart beats much more slowly than normal, and it is difficult to raise its work rate. All the body's metabolism goes into bottom gear: fat accumulates in the storage tissues, the person puts on weight, the brain slows down and the result is tiredness, disinterest and an apparent loss of intellect and ability to reason. People with low thyroid activity are often misdiagnosed as depressed.

These are all symptoms that people who have had thyroid trouble will readily recognize. Less obvious to them is the fact that low thyroid activity also affects their fat metabolism, leading to higher than normal blood cholesterol levels – and this may predispose them to heart attacks and strokes. And in children, a normal thyroxine production is essential to normal bone growth and normal sexual and intellectual development. It is vital, for example, that babies born with low thyroid function are treated immediately: delay may mean permanent loss of some intellect.

## Normal Thyroid Control Systems

So why does the thyroid go wrong? To understand how we may develop an over- or underactive thyroid, we need to know a little about the gland's control systems.

Like all hormone-secreting glands, the thyroid works on a 'feedback' system. If the amount of thyroid hormone (thyroxine) in the blood starts to fall, a 'thyroxine-detection' system sends the thyroid the message that more must be secreted. If thyroxine levels are high, no message is sent, and the thyroid obliges by secreting less hormone.

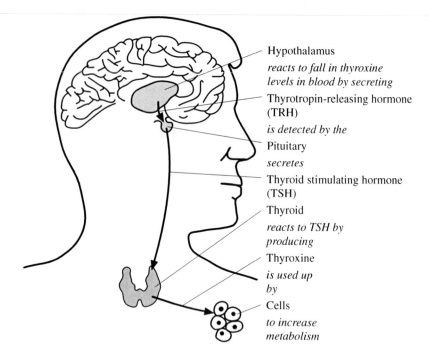

Hypothalamus
*reacts to fall in thyroxine levels in blood by secreting*
Thyrotropin-releasing hormone (TRH)
*is detected by the*
Pituitary
*secretes*
Thyroid stimulating hormone (TSH)
Thyroid
*reacts to TSH by producing*
Thyroxine
*is used up by*
Cells
*to increase metabolism*

**Regulation of thyroid secretion**

The thyroxine-detection system is in the base of the brain, in a region named the hypothalamus, which is connected by a 'stalk' to the pituitary gland. The pituitary is shaped like a sphere, rather like a large pea, and hangs just beneath the brain, in a cavity in the skull just behind the eyes and above the middle of the nose.

Cells in the hypothalamus respond to low levels of thyroxine in the blood by secreting *thyrotropin-releasing hormone*, or TRH, into special 'portal' vessels (really modified blood vessels) in the pituitary stalk. This chemical 'message' passes downwards to be picked up by cells in the front section of the pituitary gland, which respond by secreting *thyroid-stimulating hormone*, or TSH, into the bloodstream.

The normal thyroid gland is constantly reacting to changes in the levels of circulating TSH. If TSH levels are high, it pours out more thyroxine. If levels are low, the thyroid secretes less thyroxine. If there is no TSH at all (for example if the pituitary gland has been removed) the thyroid shrivels, and only produces a fraction of the thyroxine needed for normal metabolism.

To summarize: the thyroid secretes thyroxine into the bloodstream. As that 'packet' of thyroxine is used up, the levels fall. This fall is picked up by the hypothalamus, which secretes TRH that lets the pituitary gland know that more TSH is needed. The pituitary then secretes TSH, which stimulates the thyroid to produce more thyroxine.

When thyroxine levels in the bloodstream are high, the pituitary produces no TSH, and the thyroid produces no thyroxine.

## How the System Can Go Wrong

Unfortunately, although this seems a brilliant system for fine-tuning our 'acceleration' system, things can go wrong at any stage. Thyroid troubles can originate from the hypothalamus (faulty TRH secretion), from the pituitary (faulty TSH secretion), from the thyroid itself (lack of response to TSH or failure to produce thyroxine), or because the thyroid becomes 'autonomous' (the whole gland or part of the gland producing thyroxine without regard to TSH changes). So when doctors suspect a thyroid problem, the tests usually include checks on all these components of the 'hypothalamic-pituitary-thyroid' axis.

Developing normal thyroid function, therefore, depends on three organs working perfectly – the hypothalamus, the pituitary and the thyroid.

## How the Thyroid Makes Thyroxine

It's also important to understand how the thyroid gland makes and stores thyroxine, as faults in this system underlie many thyroid diseases.

Building a thyroxine molecule needs three components – iodine, thyroglobulin and thyroperoxidase.

Iodine is a 'trace' chemical element found in foods, particularly those from or growing near the sea. Our food needs to contain only tiny amounts of iodine each day to keep the thyroid gland happy. The thyroid is particularly efficient at taking iodine (in the form of iodide) up from the blood. There is normally 30 to 40 times as much iodine in thyroid tissue as in the bloodstream.

Inside the thyroid, the iodide meets up with thyroglobulin. Thyroglobulin is the protein base upon which thyroxine is synthesized: it is almost unique to the thyroid gland (though some thyroglobulin circulates in the blood).

19

Thyroperoxidase causes iodine molecules to become attached to different sites on the thyroglobulin molecule, first making molecules that contain one, then two, iodine atoms, which then 'double up' to make a molecule containing four iodine atoms. This is thyroxine, otherwise called T4 (thyroglobulin-4, because of the four iodine atoms).

However, T4 is not the complete story. While around 95 per cent of the thyroid hormone in our circulation is T4, the other 5 per cent is in the form of 'tri-iodothyronine', or T3. T3 is a thyroxine molecule that has lost one iodine atom, due to the action of 'de-iodinating' enzymes.

It turns out that T3 is between two and four times more active as a thyroid hormone than T4. Not only that, between one-third and one-half of the T4 secreted by the thyroid gland into the bloodstream is converted in the tissues into T3 by more de-iodinating enzymes. This leads most experts in thyroid disease to believe that T3 is the true thyroid hormone, and that T4 is really only a 'precursor' and a convenient way for the thyroid to store its hormone pool.

Recognizing this difference gives doctors a choice of treatment for thyroid patients in different circumstances. For most patients, T4 is the perfect answer to their problem, but for a few, T3 is preferable. Indeed, in some other cases (such as in coma – see page 94), T3 is essential. So you may be receiving thyroxine (T4) or liothyronine (T3) as your treatment. This will be discussed in more detail later on.

## Testing for Thyroid Problems

In the past, the crucial test of thyroid function was measurement of the Basal Metabolic Rate, or BMR. Before this test, the patient had to fast for several hours and be at complete rest. She would then have her oxygen use and heat production measured. This meant sitting in a climate-controlled room, being connected to tubes collecting the gases from the breath and measuring heat production in various sophisticated ways. It was a very time-consuming test involving expensive equipment.

An abnormally high BMR (high oxygen use and high heat production) meant an overactive thyroid (hyperthyroidism/thyrotoxicosis). An abnormally low BMR (low oxygen use and low heat production) meant an underactive thyroid (myxoedema).

The BMR was surprisingly accurate in diagnosing thyroid problems. In normal subjects, BMRs range from 15 per cent below the average to 5 per cent above it. Patients with an overactive thyroid have BMRs of more than 20 per cent above normal, while those with an underactive thyroid have BMRs of more than 20 per cent below the average.

However, organizing BMRs takes time, expertise and very co-operative patients – and here the word 'patient' is very appropriate. There is also the possible confusion raised by the fact that the BMR can be affected by other conditions. It is raised if the patient has a fever, certain cancers, nerve disorders or is pregnant. It is below average in the very obese and also in those suffering anorexia, during sleep, in people on beta-blocking drugs, and in people who are relatively immobile. So the BMR is more useful, once the diagnosis is made, as a pointer to how severely the thyroid problem has disturbed normal metabolism, than in making the initial diagnosis. BMR is therefore only measured nowadays in selected patients for whom this information may be useful. It is no longer a routine test for diagnosis.

Another thyroid function test which has been largely abandoned, except for very specific occasional cases, is the radio-iodine uptake test. This involves giving a tiny dose of radioactive iodine by mouth, and measuring how quickly and how much radioactivity reaches the thyroid gland. A gland that was too slow to take it up, or took up too little, was underfunctioning. However, radio-iodine tests for diagnosis are relatively unreliable: if a patient has recently taken an iodine cough medicine, this can affect results, as can drugs such as aspirin. Therefore these tests are mainly reserved today for hospital investigations in relatively unusual cases of overactive thyroid. One use, for example, is to see whether radio-iodine is taken up preferentially into a thyroid lump (nodule): more about this treatment in Chapter Five.

Today we rely for routine diagnosis largely on direct measurement from a routine blood sample of levels of the thyroid hormones T4 and T3, of TSH, and of the ability of the thyroid gland to respond normally to an injection of TRH. The results are good indicators of the likely diagnosis.

Put at its simplest, in cases of an overactive thyroid, T4 and T3 levels are abnormally high, and usually combined with a low TSH level – why this should be is explained in Chapter Three. In the case of an underactive thyroid, T4 and T3 levels are lower than normal.

The TRH injection test is then done to determine whether the problem lies with the thyroid gland itself or the pituitary control mechanism. If the TRH injection is followed by a rise in TSH in the circulation, then the pituitary is working normally and the fault is in the thyroid. If the injection fails to increase TSH levels, then the cause may be pituitary failure.

Secondary tests, used to refine a diagnosis, may include serum thyroglobulin (Tg) levels (to measure the level of thyroglobulin in the blood). These levels vary widely with different forms of hyperthyroidism. Another test measures plasma-bound iodine, which can point at times to iodine deficiency. Lack of iodine in the food and water supply – which leads to an underproduction of thyroxine – has caused much thyroid disease in the past. It is much rarer now, since most countries now recognize the importance of adding iodine to basic foods, such as salt.

Probably the single most important thyroid test is the measurement of blood levels of TSH. These levels are very low in cases of an overactive thyroid (hyperthyroidism or thyrotoxicosis) and very high in cases of an underactive thyroid (hypothyroidism or myxoedema). This test is so helpful that some experts have asked that it be used as a screening test to detect early or unsuspected thyroid disease in the general public. Up to 5 per cent of women over 50 may be identified as at risk (mainly of overactive thyroid) with the help of a routine TSH test.

While it makes sense to catch people with thyroid disease as early as possible, starting a population screening scheme – even using this relatively cheap method – would be a huge logistics problem and occupy much laboratory time, including the time and cost of recall of the many people who might be borderline positive. We are probably not yet ready for thyroid screening of the whole population here in the UK.

# Chapter Two

# How Iodine Affects the Thyroid

## Too Little Iodine

Worldwide, historically, the most common cause of thyroid disease has been lack of iodine in the diet. Without enough iodine, the thyroid gland cannot make enough thyroxine, and the person develops all the symptoms associated with an underactive thyroid, as mentioned in Chapter One. The cells in a thyroid gland starved of iodine 'over-grow' as they try to compensate for the iodine lack, so that the gland usually enlarges into what is easily recognized as a goitre.

In children born with no, or too little, thyroid activity due to a lack of iodine, the condition is called cretinism. Today to be called a cretin is highly pejorative: it is a term of abuse and no longer used in polite society, but medically speaking it is a precise diagnostic term for a person with no thyroid function because of a lack of iodine.

Cretinism leads to a loss of intellect, slower than normal growth, poor nerve and muscle co-ordination, and eventually, if left untreated, to an adult who is far below his or her potential heights, with damaged intellect, poor physical abilities and sexual immaturity. Cretinism was long a huge tragedy for some communities until the cause was found and the remedy – iodine – applied.

In the past, areas that were remote from the sea – and therefore from the most common source of iodine, in the water supply – were well known for higher than usual numbers of children with cretinism and of adults with goitres. In Britain the region most affected gave its name to the problem produced: 'Derbyshire neck'.

Lack of iodine did not always produce identical patterns of illness in different areas, however. In several remote cantons in Switzerland the lack of iodine, and therefore of thyroid activity, led particularly to deafness and an inability to speak. This 'deaf-mutism', as it was then called, rapidly declined after iodization of all table and cooking salt was introduced between 1922 and 1925.[1]

The Swiss experience is interesting, because in the same cantons there had been a long history of classical cretinism – children who, if not given iodine soon after birth, had failed to grow mentally and physically or develop into mature adults. About ten years before the iodization of salt in these cantons, the epidemic of cretinism had begun to disappear.[2] This was probably the result of better communications and education, with individual doctors and parents hearing about iodine and giving iodine supplements to the newborn. Why the 'deaf-mutism' took so much longer to eradicate is a mystery.

In the developed world, cretinism due to iodine deficiency has disappeared, because iodine is added to salt and flour, but it is still a problem in the developing world. In 1986, a study group of the Pan American Health Organization (PAHO) defined the three main features of what it called 'endemic cretinism'.[3]

1. It is associated with endemic goitre and severe iodine deficiency.
2. It is characterized by mental deficiency, with either deafness, defects in speech, disorders of standing and walking, or hypothyroidism and stunted growth.
3. Where iodine deficiency is corrected, endemic cretinism is prevented.

PAHO therefore established two distinct forms of damage due to iodine deficiency. In one, labelled 'neurological cretinism', the main problems were in controlling and co-ordinating muscles, so that the sufferers found it extremely difficult to walk or stand, along with double vision due to severe squint. In the other, labelled 'myxoedematous cretinism', there was no problem with walking but sufferers remained tiny for their age, had dry, thickened skin (the name 'myxoedema' refers to these skin changes), sparse hair and thickened nails, and did not develop sexually. The mental retardation was more severe among the neurological than the myxoedematous type, but even in the latter, it remained profound. This may be a clue to the Swiss problem: could the neurological type of iodine deficiency disease be more resistant to treatment than the myxoedemic type? Was there a missing element in those who were deaf and mute?

Some experts suggest that lack of other 'trace' elements than iodine may also play a part in thyroid failure, and that this may explain the different clinical pictures of neurological and myxoedematous cretinism. One suggestion is that lack of selenium in the water may lead to damage to the thyroid. In parts of Zaire, blood levels of selenium are lower among the population affected by cretinism than in those who are not.[4] Animal studies suggest that manganese deficiency may also play a part in goitre production.[5]

Whether or not these other trace elements are important is still a matter of argument among the experts. The general consensus remains that there is a broad spectrum of symptoms of iodine deficiency in children which ranges from the extreme neurological type to the extreme myxoedematous type, with a mixture of symptoms in between. They are just different manifestations of the same disease – low thyroid activity.

That low thyroid activity is definitely casued by an iodine deficiency is proved beyond doubt not just because iodization of salt has solved the problem, but by the experience in the Jimi Valley in New Guinea. There the local supply of rock salt from ancient sea deposits, rich in iodine, was replaced by an industrial salt low in iodine. The babies of the Jimi Valley residents began to show for the first time in their history the signs of cretinism.[6]

## 'Goitrogens'

However, there is another factor to take into account. Iodine lack is sometimes made much worse by what we eat. Some foods contain natural 'goitrogens' – chemicals that prevent iodine from being taken up by the thyroid gland or combining with thyroglobulin (see Chapter One) to make thyroxine. And that can lead to a low thyroid state with a goitre.

In Africa, cassavas make a big contribution to the daily calorie intake. They are eaten as a staple, in the same way as Europeans eat potatoes or pasta, or Eastern peoples eat rice. Unfortunately cassavas contain the goitrogen linamarin. When iodine levels are already low, but not perhaps low enough to produce cretinism in children or hypothyroidism in adults, the linamarin in cassava may tip the balance towards these illnesses. This has been proved to be the case in Zaire, where cretinism has resulted from the combination of a low iodine level and cassava consumption.[7]

Goitrogens are not exclusive to Africa nor to cassava. They were first found in plants of the Brassica family. One type of goitrogen, for example, is found in weeds growing in pastures as far apart as Tasmania and Finland.[8] This may not sound important, but the goitrogens can pass into cows' milk, and then act upon the thyroid gland of the humans who drink it.

In Europe, goitrogens from grasses have been transmitted through cows' milk not just in Finland, but also around Sheffield, in Navarre in Spain, in Bohemia (now the Czech Republic), and in the former Yugoslavia, now Croatia. Grasses and brassicas are not the only culprits: in Avila, in Spain, goitres were traced to chemicals in walnuts.

Water supplies can also contain goitrogens. *Escherichia coli*, the notorious E coli bacterium better known for food poisoning, may also produce a goitrogen. Goitres have been blamed on E coli-contaminated water supplies in Greece and West Virginia.

In mining areas, water contaminated by minerals such as phenols from shale oil and coal extraction has led to goitres in eastern Kentucky and Colombia. Chilean experts have reported goitres in areas where the water contains high levels of lithium – a chemical element that can displace iodine from the thyroxine molecule.

Goitrogens have also been found in maize, bamboo shoots, sweet potatoes and lima beans. This raises questions about the wisdom of some of the odd diets that are pushed today by various lobbyists. If you are going to go on a weird diet espousing high amounts of a particular vegetable, be certain it is safe. Any swelling of the neck in a person on a restricted diet may well be due to a goitrogen or even to iodine deficiency. The cause should be found and the diet corrected accordingly.

## Too Much Iodine

Paradoxically, the most surprising goitrogen of all is iodine itself. In 1965, it was reported that one in ten inhabitants of the Japanese island Hokkaido had goitres due to consuming excessive amounts of iodine.[9] People in the fishing villages strung along the Hokkaido coast were eating large quantities of an iodine-rich seaweed. Yet their 10 per cent goitre rate was nothing compared to the 64 per cent of children with goitres in a Chinese village, the water supply of which contained massive amounts of iodine.

So what is a safe daily intake of iodine? The recommended daily requirement of iodine is 150 micrograms. Most people in developed countries consume much more than that: in the United States the average daily iodine intake ranges from 175 to 700 micrograms.

This is much higher than the iodine content of foods a generation ago, and is mainly due to the adding of iodine to salt and bread, and the use of iodine in various forms as a food preservative. Many vitamin preparations contain 150 micrograms of iodine, so that one tablet contains all that is needed for the day, without the iodine we also consume in our food.

There are more subtle ways in which iodine gets into our food. 'Iodophors' are used as udder antiseptics in the dairy industry, and may increase, admittedly by very small amounts, the iodine content of milk. Healthfood stores promote iodine-rich foods such as kelp or dulse. There is iodine in proprietary medicines, such as cough medicines and skin creams and ointments. In the past, many children with cystic fibrosis developed goitre because the 'expectorants' – medicines to help them cough – they were taking every day contained iodine. The goitres were worst in the children who were also given sulphonamides, antibacterial agents that are also known goitrogens, interfering with the thyroid's ability to make thyroxine.

Prescription drugs can cause iodine problems, too. Amiodarone, a drug widely given to people with abnormal heart rhythms, contains 75 milligrams of iodine in each 200-milligram tablet, about 9 milligrams of the iodine being free to be absorbed into the body. This may not sound much, but remember that a milligram is a thousand micrograms, and that all you need per day is 150 micrograms.

Amiodarone may also prevent the pituitary from secreting TSH (see Chapter One). This dual action has complex effects on thyroid function, so that in some areas which are relatively deficient in iodine it can cause thyroid overactivity, and in others with plenty of natural iodine it can paradoxically block thyroid function, leading to underactivity. So if you are on amiodarone for heart problems, do consult your doctor if you start feeling unwell. Your malaise may reflect either an under- or overactive thyroid. Your doctor may well replace the amiodarone with an equivalent non-iodine-containing 'anti-arrhythmic' drug. Happily, there are plenty from which to choose.

These, however, are very specific cases of excess iodine doing harm in people particularly susceptible to such harm. It seems that for a healthy person with a normal thyroid to begin with, the extra iodine intake to which we are now exposed does no real harm. Nevertheless, when you complain for the first time of a swollen throat, and your doctor suspects this to be a goitre, you must expect to answer many questions which aim to cover all possible sources of iodine intake. Occasionally, even now, in someone who has been previously healthy, the combination of excessive iodine intake and perhaps exposure to a goitrogen may establish the cause.

# Part Two
# Explaining Thyroid Disease

# ChapterThree

# Overactive Thyroid (Hyperthyroidism)

## The Woman with Graves' Disease

There are times when the diagnosis of thyroid disease leaps out at the doctor as the patient enters the consulting room for the first time. That was the case with Jane Lang, who was 40 when she started to feel unwell. Her main complaint was that she was losing weight, in spite of her voracious appetite. She was eating twice as much as her husband, she said, yet she had lost over two stone (13 kg) in the last three months.

She had noticed, too, that she could no longer tolerate warm weather, when in previous summers she would wallow in it. And she was more irritable than before (one reason for her husband and teenage daughter pleading with her to see her doctor). She admitted to being 'nervy' and 'shaky', and that her muscles seemed weaker than before. She sweated a lot, had occasional palpitations in the daytime and had become aware, when trying to get off to sleep at night, that her heart was beating faster than it used to. Her menstrual periods were erratic, for the first time in her life. She had noticed, too, that her eyes were 'uncomfortable' and 'gritty'. She also felt that they were 'too wide open', and 'bulging' – this was a recent change, and had been the final straw that had sent her to her doctor.

Her eyes were her doctor's first clue to the diagnosis. Normally, in the relaxed position, the edges of the eyelids lie across the rims of the pupils, so that the 'whites' of the eyes (the 'sclera') are seen only at each side of the pupil. Jane's eyelids were so wide open that her pupils were surrounded by sclera, making her look as if she was staring and wild-eyed.

A quick test confirmed to her doctor that her eyes were affected by thyroid problems. He asked her to look upwards at a pen held well above her head, then to keep looking at it as he lowered it. As the eyes followed the pen downwards, the downward movement of the upper lids – which in people with normal thyroid activity move in

31

time with the eyeballs – 'lagged'. That is, there was a delay before they started to lower. They followed the eye a fraction of a second later – only a short period, but easily enough seen by the doctor. This 'lid lag' sign is a decisive confirmation of thyrotoxicosis, and shows that the overactivity of the thyroid is already causing muscle co-ordination problems.

Jane's doctor found her palm to be warm and moist. She even apologized for her 'sweaty red palms'. From her palm, her doctor turned his attention to her wrist, where her pulse was a rapid 96 beats per minute. Ten minutes later, after sitting quietly and after her natural initial anxiety at being at the surgery had died down, it was still above 90. When a sheet of paper was placed across the backs of her outstretched hands, it had a fine but very obvious 'tremor' or shake.

During the appointment minutes, Jane was never still. She fidgeted, shifted around in her chair, and tended to talk non-stop: in fact her hands, feet and whole body were never at rest. This was not just nervousness, but physical overactivity, or 'hyperactivity' – yet another sign of an overactive thyroid.

The physical examination strongly supported her doctor's initial diagnosis. Her heart rate, even at the end of the consultation, when she had been reassured and seated for more than 20 minutes, remained well above 90 beats per minute. Her blood pressure was slightly raised, at 150/95 millimetres mercury (mm/Hg) (the norm is around 120/80 mm Hg).

Jane's muscles and reflexes were abnormal, too. Tapping the tendons at the elbows, wrists, knees and ankles with a small rubber hammer gave rise to exaggerated responses. The forearms, hands, lower legs and feet responded far faster and more positively than normal, and the feet even went into a series of jerks when the Achilles tendons were 'tapped'. When these excessive reflex responses were found to go along with quite severe loss of muscle power (she had a very poor grip even with her stronger hand, and her arm and leg muscles were much weaker than normal), the clinical diagnosis of an overactive thyroid was complete.

The next step was to examine her thyroid gland. Although Jane had not noticed it herself, it was enlarged. Her doctor found it to be swollen, marginally firmer than normal, the right side being perhaps slightly more enlarged than the left. It wasn't knobbly, and it wasn't tender. She did not complain of any pain in the throat, even when fairly firm pressure was applied to it. When the doctor placed a stethoscope over the larger right lobe, he could hear a slight rushing sound – the 'bruit' referred to in Chapter One.

The examination was completed with blood tests. Off to the lab were sent requests for venous blood thyroxine and TSH levels (see Chapter One).

In the meantime, Jane was advised that she probably had the Graves' disease form of overactive thyroid (thyrotoxicosis), and that this would almost certainly be confirmed by the blood tests, the results of which would be available in a few days. It was explained to her that all her symptoms were being caused by the fact that her thyroid gland was secreting too much thyroid hormone into the bloodstream, mostly in the form of thyroxine, and that her treatment would aim to reverse that process.

It was also explained that there were three main treatment options open to her and her doctors – tablets to reduce the thyroxine production, radio-iodine to destroy the thyroid's ability to produce thyroxine, and surgery to reduce the enlarged thyroid mass, so that the remnant of the gland would produce less. These three types of treatment, and the reasons for and against them, are described in more detail in Chapter Five.

To begin with, her doctor prescribed an anti-thyroid drug, as a daily tablet, but he also arranged for her to see a specialist in thyroid disease to examine the best long-term treatment options for her. Jane was reasonably happy with this, and one week later she returned to say that she was already feeling much better.

After that week of treatment, her resting heart rate was down to a steady 72 beats per minute. Her hands were no longer hot and sweaty. She could tolerate the warm weather better, her family had found she was much less agitated and irritable, and she herself knew she was quieter and found it easier to relax. She was sleeping better at night she was eating more sensibly and had put on nearly two pounds (1 kg) in weight, although she was still more than a stone (6 kg) underweight. She was looking forward to her appointment with the consultant with confidence, rather than with apprehension. Her family could not believe her mental and physical improvement.

This was just the start for Jane. Over the next year she continued to improve. She is now at the correct weight for her height, and is back to her old normal self. Her doctor can no longer feel her thyroid gland. The drug dose appears to have been just right, as her blood tests show normal levels of thyroxine and TSH. Her consultant is now considering taking her off her drug to see if her disease is in 'remission' – a period in which the thyroid can work normally again and will not slip back into a hyper-productive state. The chances are good that Jane will remain 'euthyroid' – in a normal thyroid state – once the treatment stops. Graves' disease is one which does vary, with periods of excess activity interspersed with normal activity. It is hoped that the treatment has helped to coax Jane's thyroid into a remission, but she will always need to be followed up, using blood tests, so as to nip in the bud any return to florid Graves' disease.

Happily, Jane's eyes are also gradually improving. They are less prominent now, and she can close her eyelids more easily than before. She still wears sunglasses when outside in bright daylight, partly because her eyes are still a little sensitive to light, and partly to protect them from wind and dust.

This is probably the appropriate place to explain why this particular form of thyroid disease is called Graves' disease, and what we now know about it.

R J Graves was a London doctor who in 1835 reported in his lectures in the *London Medical and Surgical Journal* on three patients with palpitations and swellings of the thyroid. There was also a fourth 'whose eyeballs were so enlarged that when she slept or tried to close her eyes the lids were incapable of closing, and when she was awake her eyes showed the white sclerotic all around the cornea'.[1]

Five years later, C A von Basedow described a series of patients with all the symptoms of an overactive thyroid (thyrotoxicosis) in a German medical journal.[2] To this day, thyrotoxicosis is described in Britain as Graves' disease, and on the Continent as von Basedow's disease. Actually neither should get the credit: it should really be called Parry's disease.

Caleb Parry was a British (probably Welsh) doctor who, practising in Bath in 1786, saw five patients with heart failure linked to swelling in the thyroid area. One had 'a remarkable extrusion of the globes (eyes) from the socket'. His papers were not published until 1825, after his death, but he certainly has prior claim to the recognition that thyroid disease was linked to heart and eye problems.[3]

Graves' disease usually starts between the ages of 20 and 50 years, but it can occur at any age. It can start slowly, then progress, or all the symptoms can 'burst out' at once. The experts still argue about whether or not it follows sudden unexpected stress, such as a serious accident or infection, bereavement or a psychological problem. Some link it with severe dieting and anorexia.

One study that looked into the past stresses of people with and without Graves' disease did not show a difference between them.[4]

Graves' disease, like Hashimoto's thyroiditis (see Chapter Four), does run in families. If one identical twin develops it, the other has between a 30 and 60 per cent chance of developing it as well. This is in contrast to the 3 to 9 per cent chance in non-identical twins – a difference that is a powerful argument for a strong inherited (genetic) component in the illness.

However, the fact that the rate for both identical twins having the disease is not 100 per cent after one twin develops it proves that there must be another, non-inherited component. We have yet to find it.

## Hyperthyroidism without Graves' Disease

Mary Brown, like Jane Lang, also had an overactive thyroid, but it was far more difficult to spot. Widowed just a year before, at the age of 59, she had no eye signs, had not lost weight, did not feel anxious or shaky, and could tolerate the heat as well as anyone else. Her main complaint was simply tiredness. She was tired all the time, and became breathless on the slightest exertion, something that was quite new to her.

But what took her to the doctor (she didn't like bothering him about her tiredness, which she put down to depression after the loss of her husband) was a bout of fluttering in her chest, late at night, that frightened her. It disappeared on its own, but a visit to her doctor the next morning showed that her heartbeat was erratic. There were runs of faster and slower beats, so that it was difficult to count accurately how many beats there were each minute.

Mary's doctor, who knew her well, found this curious, because only a year before, at the Well Woman clinic, her heart had been normal.

He thought that she might have had a 'silent' heart attack – a heart attack without pain – that had left her with a damaged heart muscle, so he ordered an electrocardiogram, along with blood tests for anaemia and thyroid function. He knew that one possibility in an older woman whose heartbeat becomes erratic (the term is atrial fibrillation) is an overactive thyroid.

The ECG was clear for heart damage – she had not had a heart attack. But the erratic heartbeat remained. Her thyroid tests (high T4 and T3 levels) confirmed that Mary had an overactive thyroid. Her doctor referred her immediately to the local thyroid specialist, who arranged for treatment. Within two weeks, she had not only lost her erratic heartbeat: she was feeling much better, less tired and less breathless. She was able to stop her anti-thyroid drug. Over the next few months she improved further. Her only problem was that, after six months, her blood tests revealed that she was becoming hypothyroid (her T4 and T3 levels were too low).

Mary is now taking a low dose of thyroxine every day. This is keeping her feeling and looking fine. In her own words, she is a 'new woman'.

## Explaining Jane's and Mary's Illnesses

So how did Jane and Mary come to develop an overactive thyroid? Although their illnesses were so different, they probably shared the same underlying problem.

As explained in Chapter One, the normal thyroid reacts to thyroid-stimulating hormone (TSH) produced by the pituitary gland by forming thyroxine and secreting it into the bloodstream. The rise in blood thyroxine levels is picked up by the hypothalamus, which then 'switches off' its production of thyrotropin-releasing hormone (TRH). The lack of TRH arriving at the pituitary in turn switches off the production and secretion of TSH, to which the thyroid responds by shutting down its thyroxine 'production line'.

The consequent lower blood levels of thyroxine are then 'picked up' by the hypothalamus, which responds by secreting TRH. This stimulates the pituitary to secrete TSH, causing the thyroid to secrete more thyroxine – and the cycle continues.

Things can go wrong at each stage of this feedback cycle, and this chapter explains how they can do so, and how they lead to an over- or underactive thyroid. It also explains how understanding these failures has led to very effective treatment for them.

First, however, a word about goitres, or thyroid swellings. The fact that a thyroid gland has enlarged, so that it is easy to see and feel, has no bearing at all on whether it is overactive, underactive or putting out normal amounts of thyroxine. The thyroid may have enlarged in response to a lack of iodine, and still be underactive because it is producing too little thyroxine. It may have enlarged because it is responding to an excess of TSH, or is responding excessively to normal levels of TSH, or is just churning out thyroxine at high levels independently of TSH levels. In all these cases it will be hyperactive.

However, the enlargement may be just enough to produce exactly the right amount of thyroxine for the body's needs, in which case the person is described in medical terms as 'euthyroid' – neither hyper- nor hypo-thyroid. Or it may have enlarged as a result of an inflammation or 'auto-immune' reaction (to be explained later in this chapter): in such cases the thyroid problem may have started as one of over-activity, but ended as underactivity (hypothyroidism).

If swelling of the thyroid gives little information on whether the thyroid is over- or underactive, then the same goes for thyroids that can't be felt or seen at all. People can be hyperthyroid or hypothyroid, yet have no visible or palpable thyroid swelling.

So, although examining the thyroid can be an important pointer to the diagnosis of thyroid disease, it isn't necessarily a guide to what is going on inside it.

## Overactive Thyroid – Hyperthyroidism and Thyrotoxicosis

The term hyperthyroidism simply means an overactive thyroid, one that is constantly producing too much thyroxine (T4) and tri-iodothyronine (T3) (see Chapter One). It has three main causes:

1. An excess of TSH is reaching the gland, causing it to produce too much thyroxine.
2. Some other substance in the blood is acting upon the thyroid gland in exactly the same way as TSH.
3. Part of the thyroid gland is acting 'autonomously', out of the control of TSH, so that it is constantly producing too much thyroxine.

Around 60 per cent of all cases of hyperthyroidism take the form of 'thyrotoxicosis'. Strictly, thyrotoxicosis is the name for the illness caused by hyperthyroidism. However, some people with an overactive thyroid do not show the complete set of symptoms that mark out people with thyrotoxicosis (they do not appear 'toxic'), so the two terms (hyperthyroidism and thyrotoxicosis) are not completely interchangeable.

In most people with thyrotoxicosis (see earlier in this chapter for a description of a typical case), the second explanation for its cause holds true. Their thyroids are constantly being stimulated to produce excessive amounts of thyroxine by a substance other than TSH. In fact, TSH levels are lower than normal in most thyrotoxic patients. This paradox (one would expect high levels of TSH in people whose thyroid glands are over-producing thyroxine) began to be explained as long ago as 1956. Then, New Zealanders D D Adams and H D Purves discovered a substance, not TSH itself, in the blood of many thyrotoxic patients which stimulated the thyroid of guinea pigs for much longer than did TSH.[5] They called this substance LATS – standing for Long Acting Thyroid Stimulator.

LATS has since been renamed thyroid-stimulating antibody (TSAb) or thyroid-stimulating immunoglobulin (TSI). We know now that it is produced by the body as a result of a problem in the immune system. Most people with thyrotoxicosis have what is defined by doctors as an 'auto-immune disease'. To understand what this is, you need to know a little about the immune system, how it works, and how it can go wrong.

### The Immune System

Our immune system is our main line of defence against infections, 'foreign proteins' and cancers. Its aim is to recognize any potential illness-inducing foreign substances and to neutralize them before harm can be done. It has two main components: white blood cells ('lymphocytes' and 'macrophages') and circulating 'immunoglobulins'.

Explained simply, the immunoglobulins are complex protein substances which, aided by the lymphocytes, target the foreign proteins, and latch on to their surfaces. Once 'coated' with an immunoglobulin, the foreign material is now recognizable to the macrophages, which engulf it and destroy it. In brief, the immunoglobulins are 'antibodies' that are formed to attack the 'antigens', the proteins on the surface of the germs that have provoked the immune response in the first place.

The system works well, for example against infection-causing bacteria and viruses. The antigenic proteins on their surfaces, being non-human, are instantly recognized as being 'foreign', and the lymphocytes, immunoglobulin antibodies and macrophages work together to destroy them.

The same goes for cancer cells. The changes in chemistry that make cancer cells different from normal cells are assumed by the body to be antigens. They are identified by the immune system as such, and immunoglobulin antibodies are raised against them. By almost exactly the same process as with bacteria and viruses, the newly formed cancer cells are picked out for destruction by this combination of white blood cells and the circulating protective antibody immunoglobulin proteins. The process is happening all through life: it is only when this 'seek and destroy' immune system mechanism eventually fails that cancer cells manage to multiply.

The immune system works in the same way to tackle non-infectious and non-cancerous foreign proteins, too. The most obvious of these are the proteins (again, antigens) on the surface of pollen grains. We inhale millions of them each summer, and more than 85 per cent of us never give them a thought. That's because when our immune system destroys the pollen molecules in our eyes, noses, throats and chests, they do so by the usual antigen-antibody reaction without producing a new set of irritating chemicals.

The other 15 per cent of us, however, have cause to complain about their body's reaction to pollens. In targeting and trying to neutralize them, an 'allergic' reaction is produced. Instead of the antibody-antigen interaction running smoothly, and the offending foreign material being quietly disposed of, other chemicals are released into the tissues. These chemicals, the best known of which is histamine (but there are several others), are released into the tissues in the eyes, nose, throat and lungs. This produces the red, itchy eyes, the irritated, stuffy, runny nose, and the sneezing of hay fever in some people, and the wheeze and breathlessness of asthma in others.

This process is a true allergy. If we have the wrong genetic make-up, the antigens of pollens (and of other substances such as house dust mite, and perhaps the dust from feathers) become allergens.

Most people are blissfully unaware of the hard work our immune systems are doing every minute of our lives to keep us healthy. People with allergies are only too aware that their immune systems have gone wrong.

What has this to do with thyrotoxicosis? Simply that here, too, the immune system has gone wrong. And here, too, a little explanation is needed.

For thyroid-stimulating hormone (TSH) to carry the message to the thyroid gland to manufacture more thyroxine, it has to latch on to 'receptors' on the surface of the thyroid cells. The process is something like a jigsaw. The receptors for TSH on the thyroid cell surfaces have a particular shape, and the circulating TSH molecules from the pituitary gland have a mirror-image shape that fits them precisely. So precisely, in fact, that TSH molecules will not fit on to the surface of any other protein on any other cell surface in the body. Once the TSH has attached to its thyroid cell receptor, the cell is stimulated to produce thyroxine.

This effect lasts only a few hours, before other chemical systems break down the bond between TSH and its receptor, freeing the receptor to receive future TSH molecules as they arrive. While there is no TSH attached to the thyroid cell surface, the cell lapses into its quiet mode, and releases no further thyroxine. Only when the next TSH molecule comes along is the thyroxine production and secretion stepped up again. When this system is working normally, it ensures that just enough thyroxine is produced, no more nor less than required.

Unfortunately in thyrotoxicosis, the system is no longer working normally. For some reason, still obscure, the immune system sees the TSH receptor protein on the surface of the thyroid cells as a 'foreign antigen'. It therefore raises a circulating antibody – an immune globulin – to the TSH receptor protein. This antibody, the TSAb mentioned on page 38, is shaped just like TSH, so that it acts like TSH, stimulating the cells to produce thyroxine.

However, the antibody differs from TSH in a very important way: it remains attached to the cell for far longer, and is resistant to the body's efforts to split it from the cell surface. So the cell continues to make thyroxine for far longer than it needs.

The excess thyroxine that is secreted into the bloodstream is equivalent to a stuck accelerator, and the body can't find a way to take the foot off the pedal. The hypothalamus reacts to the rising thyroxine levels by shutting down production of thyrotropin-releasing hormone (TRH). The pituitary responds by lowering TSH production. But the thyroid cells, stuck on 'go', can't heed the message to brake, and keep on churning out thyroxine.

This process, in which the body 'sees' part of its own normal tissues as a foreign protein and makes an antibody to it, is called auto-immune disease. The thyroid is not the only organ that can be affected by auto-immune changes: it happens in some forms of arthritis, when antibodies are raised to the tissues that form the surfaces of joints, and in types of anaemia and chronic bowel disease.

### Why Do People Develop Auto-Immune Diseases?

Why should people suddenly be struck down by an auto-immune disease in adulthood? Two factors apparently need to be present. The first is an inherited tendency to develop the disease. Studies of the different types of white blood cell in people with and without thyroid disease strongly suggest that there is an inherited defect in a group of cells called 'suppressor T-lymphocytes'. To go into detail on the science behind the different types of white blood cells is well beyond the remit of this book. Suffice it to state here that normal suppressor T-lymphocytes help to prevent the immune system from mistaking our own proteins as 'foreign'. Lack of efficient T-lymphocytes could easily, in theory, induce auto-immune disease.

However, we only need to mobilize our suppressor T-lymphocyte activity in emergencies, such as times when our immune system is in danger of being overwhelmed. These times include severe infections and injuries (such as with burns or road accidents), or exposure to certain drugs, or even mental stress, such as sudden unexpected bereavement. The immune system tends to become less efficient as we grow older, so that although most people susceptible to thyrotoxicosis start life with an adequate T-lymphocyte system they become much more likely to develop it from their twenties onwards. Nevertheless, thyrotoxicosis can also start in childhood.

Some backing for this theory is offered by the fact that many people date the start of their thyrotoxicosis from a short time after some other serious illness, accident or mental stress. It has been reported as starting after women have gone on an extreme diet, amounting almost to starvation. It is relatively common in women who have had anorexia nervosa.

Not all experts agree that stress can lead to thyrotoxicosis. J Gray and R Hoffenberg, writing in 1985, found that the number and severity of stresses experienced by people with thyrotoxicosis did not differ from those in people with normal thyroids.[6] In reply, R Volpe, writing in 1991, felt that Gray and Hoffenberg had not taken the genetic immune vulnerability to thyrotoxicosis of the thyroid patients into account: he is convinced that there is a relationship between stress and the start of thyrotoxicosis.[7]

Of course, if you have thyrotoxicosis, whether or not stress was the incident that started it off is probably now immaterial to you. What you want to know is how the illness normally progresses once it has started. This is explained more fully earlier in this chapter, where typical cases of thyrotoxicosis are described. It is enough to state here that it is a 'remitting and relapsing' disease, which even if untreated often waxes and wanes. It seems that the change in the immune system is not necessarily permanent, and that the auto-immune process can switch itself off. So management often aims at 'cooling off' the thyroid overactivity until it starts to settle: if it shows no signs of doing so, then treatments to deal permanently with thyroid overactivity can then be undertaken. These treatments are described in Chapter Five.

## Other Causes of Overactive Thyroid

As mentioned above, most people with thyrotoxicosis have an auto-immune cause for their problem. Their high blood levels of thyroxine are combined with low or even totally absent TSH levels, because their hypothalamus and pituitary are working normally and respond to the high thyroid hormone levels by shutting down TRH and TSH production. Their feedback mechanisms are intact, but there is an intruder, in the form of auto-immune antibody, that spoils the picture.

### Pituitary Problems

However, some people with hyperthyroidism have both high TSH and high thyroxine levels. In their case, the fundamental problem is not in the thyroid itself, but in the pituitary gland. The pituitary keeps on sending out the signal (TSH) to the thyroid to push more thyroxine into the bloodstream, despite there being too much thyroxine there already. The 'feedback' system is not working.

This is called 'thyrotropin-induced hyperthyroidism' or TSH-induced hyperthyroidism. It has also been labelled 'inappropriate TSH secretion' disease.

TSH-induced hyperthyroidism is caused by one of two faults. Either there is a small tumour in the pituitary that constantly secretes TSH, out of the control of the feedback system, or the pituitary gland is resistant to the 'shut down' message that high circulating thyroid hormone levels bring to it. It then continues to secrete TSH regardless.

Hyperthyroidism due to pituitary tumour is relatively rare. In fact, the first definitely diagnosed case was reported only in 1970, by C R Hamilton and colleagues.[8] By 1991, only just over 100 cases had been described in the medical journals.

In the early days, such pituitary tumours were not detected until they were fairly large and difficult to treat, so that they could be lethal. Today, whenever hyperthyroidism is the suspected diagnosis, the combination of high TSH and high thyroid hormone levels in the blood is the prime indicator for a search for a pituitary problem. Sophisticated X-rays and scans of the skull, along with certain bio-chemical tests for the presence of a TSH-secreting pituitary tumour, clinch the diagnosis even at the very earliest stages, when the tumours are microscopic and have not grown enough to be detected on X-ray.

**Thyroid Hormone Resistance**

Hyperthyroidism due to 'thyroid hormone resistance' needs a little more explanation here. In the usual form of thyroid hormone resistance, all the organs are resistant to the effects of the two main thyroid hormones, T4 and T3. In other words, they need much higher than normal amounts of the hormones to react. For the heart to go faster, the muscles to act more energetically, the brain to think faster, the metabolism to tick over faster, the thyroid must produce much more than the normal amounts of hormone.

So people with thyroid hormone resistance have persistently higher than normal blood levels of T4 and T3, and usually normal, or perhaps slightly raised TSH levels. Giving them extra thyroxine fails to speed up the heart or general physical activity or metabolism, and does not lower the pituitary's secretion of TSH.

Most people with thyroid hormone resistance seem outwardly to be perfectly normal. Their extra output of thyroid hormones keeps them 'euthyroid' (neither 'hyper' nor 'hypo') and they may only be diagnosed as being thyroid hormone resistant by a chance finding of their high levels on a routine blood count. Many cases, however, are found because the patients' thyroid glands have enlarged (to cope with the need for higher hormone output), so that they develop a goitre.

However, a small proportion of people with thyroid hormone resistance show it almost exclusively in the pituitary. That is, the pituitary is less sensitive than, say, the heart to the effects of thyroid hormone. This is 'selective pituitary thyroid hormone resistance'. This means that, in the presence of normal thyroid hormone levels, the pituitary continues to send out high levels of TSH to the thyroid gland, which then secretes more hormone. The heart reacts to this normally by speeding up, and the other organs follow suit. This leads to the person developing the classical symptoms of an overactive thyroid, with normal levels of TSH and high levels of circulating thyroid hormone.

Obviously the various types of hyperthyroidism must be treated very differently. In the usual form of auto-immune thyrotoxicosis (Graves' disease), in which the pituitary is normal, the aim is to quieten down the thyroid activity, usually using drugs. In TSH-induced hyperthyroidism (due to a tumour or to pituitary thyroid hormone resistance) the aim is to lessen the signal from the pituitary that induces the thyroid overactivity.

When there is a pituitary tumour, it may be removed surgically or by radiotherapy. When the problem is selective pituitary thyroid hormone resistance, then the usual choice is a combination of beta-blocking drugs and small daily doses of T3. The beta-blockers slow the heartbeat, while the pituitary reacts to the T3 (the pituitary is often more sensitive to T3 levels than to T4). Surgery and radiotherapy to the pituitary are not options for people with pituitary thyroid hormone resistance, as these treatments would destroy other important pituitary functions, and produce more problems than they would solve.

If a patient with TSH-induced hyperthyroidism is mistakenly diagnosed as having Graves' disease (auto-immune thyrotoxicosis), and treated accordingly, there can be serious consequences. First, if the cause is a tumour, it may continue to grow, so that the mass inside the head can start pressing on vital organs, such as the optic nerves leading into the brain from the eyes. This causes disturbances in vision which can lead to blindness if unchecked. It also causes headaches, as pressure builds up in the brain.

Sadly, sometimes the true diagnosis only comes to light after the person is treated for thyrotoxicosis by 'thyroid ablation' – removal of most of the thyroid either by surgery or by radiation (radio-iodine). The normal thyroid gland (and it is normal in people with TSH-induced hyperthyroidism) often re-grows very quickly, and the symptoms of hyperthyroidism reappear. Only then does the penny drop and a pituitary cause is sought. Hopefully, today such mistakes are rare, as doctors are now very much aware of the importance of blood levels of both TSH and thyroid hormones.

It is vital, therefore, for doctors to distinguish between hyperthyroidism due to auto-immune disease (Graves' disease) and that due to TSH-induced disease. There are clues in the symptoms themselves.

TSH-induced hyperthyroidism (due to tumour or to pituitary thyroid hormone resistance) and Graves' disease both produce a smooth goitre and the usual fast heartbeat, raging appetite and weight loss. TSH-induced hyperthyroidism does not, however, produce the more obvious eye signs. And about one in three people with TSH-induced hyperthyroidism due to tumour have other hormone problems, too, linked to abnormal pituitary function. As pituitary feedback systems also involve the control of sex hormone output from the ovaries and testicles, there can be a loss of sexual drive and changes in the menstrual cycle.

In contrast to auto-immune thyrotoxicosis (Graves' disease), in which women sufferers outnumber men by between five and ten to one, TSH-induced hyperthyroidism affects men and women equally. So a man showing features of hyperthyroidism should have pituitary investigations as a routine.

Most people are between 30 and 60 years old before a pituitary tumour produces symptoms such as an overactive thyroid, although it has been reported in someone as young as 17.[9] The tendency to the other form of pituitary hyperthyroidism, thyroid hormone resistance, is inherited, so that people with it may remember close relatives with goitres, but who may not have been diagnosed as being hyperthyroid, and may even have had myxoedema (see Chapter Four).

## The 'Hot Nodule' Thyroid

As if the above causes of hyperthyroidism weren't enough, there is still another form of it that needs to be mentioned. This is the thyroid with 'hot nodules'.

The thyroid produces thyroid hormone in microscopic structures called 'follicles' – tiny spheres which collect the hormone inside them, to be extruded when the message of high thyroid-stimulating hormone (TSH) levels reaches them from the bloodstream. In the normal thyroid, these follicles remain their normal size and obey the 'feedback' rules explained above. While TSH levels are low, they make no more thyroid hormone; when TSH levels are high, they make more thyroid hormone and secrete it into the circulation. The follicles are all of similar, uniform size, and this makes the surface of the normal thyroid smooth and unremarkable.

However, in some people, some of their follicles don't respond to the 'brake' of low TSH, and they continue to make thyroid hormone regardless. In these cases, the follicles become bigger and much more active than the rest of the thyroid tissue. These overactive follicles may cluster together to produce multiple 'nodules' of overactive ('hot') thyroid tissue. And they can produce enough of an excess of thyroid hormone to produce the symptoms of hyperthyroidism (overactive thyroid).

The hot nodule process is very slow, so that this type of hyperthyroidism develops slowly over several years, usually in older people who have had goitres for many years, but who have never before shown any thyroid symptoms – the sharp contrast with Graves' disease (which starts abruptly and is usually linked to a 'smooth' thyroid, rather than a nodular one) was reported for the first time by the American doctor H S Plummer as long ago as 1913.[10] It has been called Plummer's disease, after him.

The people most likely to develop a 'hot nodule' hyperthyroidism are older women who have had a goitre for ten years or more, but who have only recently started to feel unwell. The predominant symptoms are a fast irregular pulse, palpitations, weight loss, depression, anxiety and insomnia. Their TSH levels are usually low, but their thyroid hormone (T3 and T4) levels are high (because the nodules are producing them in spite of the low levels of TSH).

Very occasionally, multi-nodular goitres with hyperthyroidism occur in younger people, mostly in their thirties. In these cases it affects men and women in roughly equal proportion.

The aim of treatment of both types of 'hot nodule' hyperthyroidism is to remove the offending thyroid tissue. For the younger group this is usually by surgery, for the older group radio-iodine therapy is usually chosen (see Chapter Five).

There is a final group of people with a single hot nodule in their thyroid. The specialists define these single nodules as 'autonomously functioning thyroid nodules' or AFTNs. Scans of these patients' thyroid glands show a single area of thyroid hormone over-production. AFTNs are more common in areas where iodine levels in the water, soil and food are naturally low. Nowadays they are relatively rare, but they need to be recognized because a small proportion of them are cancerous. So it is usual for people with them to have a 'fine-needle aspiration biopsy' (which uses a syringe and needle to take material out of the centre of the nodule for testing) to rule out more serious disease.

Treatment of AFTNs has the same aim as that of the other forms of hot nodules – to remove the abnormal thyroid tissue. This is more easily done when there is a single AFTN, which can often be removed without disturbing the rest of the thyroid gland, leaving the person with normal thyroid function. This can be done either surgically or by a finely measured dose of radio-iodine, more of which is taken up by the AFTN than by the normal thyroid cells.

## 'Thyroiditis': Silent and Subacute

A chapter on the causes of hyperthyroidism would not be complete without mention of 'thyroiditis'. The suffix 'itis' is generally taken to mean an inflammation, so that tonsillitis is an inflammation of the tonsils, and appendicitis an inflammation of the appendix, and so on. Most inflammations are assumed to be caused by an infectious agent, such as a virus or bacterium.

Thyroiditis is a convenient word, therefore, for an illness that appears to be caused by an inflammation of the thyroid gland, which usually comes to a peak then dies away, hopefully leaving the person with a normal thyroid. We recognize two forms of it – 'silent thyroiditis' and 'subacute thyroiditis'.

## Silent Thyroiditis

Silent, or painless, thyroiditis is – or perhaps it is better to say was – a strange disease that was diagnosed fairly often in the late 1970s and early 1980s, but seems to have waned recently. Clusters of cases in a particular district or at a particular time of year suggested to researchers that it may be caused by a viral infection, but exhaustive blood tests for any evidence of viruses have failed to find them.

Women with silent thyroiditis only outnumber men with it by less than two to one, so that it is different from the usual thyrotoxicosis, and most sufferers are in their young or middle adult lives.

Silent thyroiditis causes the usual general symptoms of an overactive thyroid, with fast resting pulse and loss of weight despite eating well. But it also produces more unusual symptoms such as an erratic heartbeat ('atrial fibrillation'), widespread muscle pains and even temporary muscle paralysis. When it hits a woman just after childbirth it is strongly linked with depression. It does not cause the bulging eyes ('exophthalmos') and skin myxoedema (thickening) seen in standard cases of thyrotoxicosis.

In silent thyroiditis the gland itself is usually around twice or three times larger than normal, but it is not tender or painful. The thyrotoxic (hyperthyroid) phase lasts about four to eight weeks, then subsides, leaving most people with normal thyroid function. About four in ten people with it then become hypothyroid (develop an underactive thyroid – see Chapter Four); if this phase lasts more than six months, it is usually permanent.

Silent thyroiditis is differentiated from Graves' disease by blood tests. The inflamed gland seems less able to take up iodine from the bloodstream than normal, so that if thyroiditis is suspected a 'radioiodine uptake test' is done. The thyroid gland affected by Graves' disease avidly takes up much more radio-iodine than normal; in silent thyroiditis, its iodine uptake is very low. (See Chapter One for a description of the radio-iodine uptake test.)

The next step is to perform a 'fine needle biopsy' of the gland. This involves removing a tiny piece of the gland under local anaesthetic. Under the microscope, the thyroid in silent thyroiditis shows many 'lymphocytes' – white blood cells that are part of the body's anti-inflammatory response. The thyroid in Graves' disease does not contain any excess of white blood cells.

Once the diagnosis has been made, how to treat it becomes the problem. The general consensus on silent thyroiditis is 'masterly inactivity'. If the symptoms are not too annoying, most people can be reassured that they will settle in 8 to 12 weeks. Beta-blockers may be given for the fast heart rate, and perhaps a sedative for the overactivity (and even a tranquillizer for anxiety), but no anti-thyroid drugs are given (see Chapter Five for treatments of an overactive thyroid). If the condition is more severe, the inflammation may be treated with a short sharp course of a cortisone-like steroid, such as prednisolone.

Once the illness has subsided, people with silent thyroiditis need to be followed for several years, as about half of them eventually develop thyroid problems (usually an underactive thyroid). About one in ten may have further episodes of silent thyroiditis.

*Subacute Thyroiditis*
Subacute thyroiditis has a host of other names, including granulomatous thyroiditis, giant cell thyroiditis, creeping thyroiditis and de Quervain's thyroiditis. This last is because of the description of the disease by Dr F de Quervain in 1904.[11] It should be more fairly called Mygind's disease, because of the earlier description of it by Dr H Mygind in 1895.[12]

Unlike the lack of evidence for any link between silent thyroiditis and viral infections, subacute thyroiditis does often follow a cold or flu-like illness, or summer diarrhoea (an infection with enteroviruses). Just before the thyroid symptoms begin, the patient develops muscle aches and pains, feels generally unwell and is very tired. Studies of viral antibodies in the blood have linked it with mumps, measles, influenza, the common cold, Epstein-Barr virus (which causes glandular fever), Coxsackie virus (thought at one time to be linked also to myalgic encephalopathy, or ME) and cat-scratch fever. However, none of these associations has been proved beyond doubt, and the cause of most cases remains unknown.

People with subacute thyroiditis usually have neck pain and a tender thyroid gland – again pointers to the fact that they do not have Graves' disease. About half have recently had a cold. The pain may be in only one side of the thyroid, or involve the whole gland, and it often spreads to the angle of the jaw and towards the ear on the same side as the thyroid pain. The ear pain can be so bad that the doctor can mistake the condition for an ear infection, and miss the thyroid problem. (This is one reason for trainee doctors being taught always to examine the thyroid gland in people complaining of earache – a piece of advice sometimes forgotten in a busy GP clinic.)

Less often the pain is worst in the upper chest or inside the throat. Wherever the pain is worst, it is made worse still by coughing, swallowing, turning the head or by wearing tight neckwear such as a tie or buttoned collar. Even gentle touching of the gland, as in a doctor's examination, can be very painful.

Other symptoms include fever, muscle pains, loss of appetite, nervousness, trembling, intolerance to warmth and a fast resting heartbeat. The thyroid is usually enlarged and firm, and very tender. Although the throat can be very sore, there are no glands in the neck (as would be expected with tonsillitis). With all these symptoms, the person looks and feels generally ill and is obviously flushed.

Subacute thyroiditis usually lasts around three to four months, although it can continue for up to a year. People enduring the longer illness have a persistently painful and tender enlarged thyroid, the discomfort outlasting the symptoms of the overactive thyroid, which usually subside within four to ten weeks. As with silent thyroiditis, a few people with subacute thyroiditis become hypothyroid (develop an underactive thyroid) for a few months. Interestingly, despite the fact that subacute thyroiditis is a much more severe illness than silent thyroiditis, many fewer 'subacute' than 'silent' patients go on to develop thyroid disease afterwards.

As with other forms of hyperthyroidism, making the diagnosis often depends on the blood test results. There are high blood levels of T4 and T3, thyroglobulin and iodine, and low levels of thyroid-stimulating hormone (TSH). As in silent thyroiditis, the radio-iodine uptake by the gland is low. One test that is strongly positive is the 'ESR', or erythrocyte sedimentation rate. This is the speed with which red blood cells settle out from the plasma in a column of blood, and it is an accurate reflection of how active the inflammation is. The normal ESR range is from around 1 to 9 millimetres per hour. In subacute thyroiditis, it is common for the ESR to be as high as 100 mm per hour. If the ESR is normal in a suspected case of subacute thyroiditis, this should spark a search for another diagnosis. A newer test for inflammation, C-reactive protein, or CRP, reveals similar abnormalities. Fine-needle aspiration biopsy confirms the diagnosis, when this is needed, by the typical appearance of inflammation (white blood cells and excessive fluid) under the microscope.

The treatment of subacute thyroiditis can be spectacularly success-ful. Cortisone-like steroids such as prednisolone relieve the neck pain and tenderness within 24 hours. In fact, if they do not do so the diagnosis should be reconsidered. The hyperthyroidism (overac-tive thyroid) usually subsides along with the symptoms of the inflam-mation. It is usual to start with a high dose of prednisolone, then taper it off so that the whole course does not last more than four weeks. In the very rare patient whose pain and tenderness do not respond, most of the thyroid gland may have to be removed by sur-gery or by radio-iodine therapy (see Chapter Five).

# Chapter Four

# Underactive Thyroid (Hypothyroidism)

An underactive thyroid (hypothyroidism) may seem to be simply the opposite of an overactive thyroid (hyperthyroidism), but the two states, although opposite in effect on the body's metabolism and very different in the symptoms they cause, are not mutually exclusive in each person. Some thyroid illnesses may start off as hyperthyroidism, then develop into hypothyroidism. And people who have had their overactive thyroid glands treated (by surgery or radio-iodine – see Chapter Five) may lapse into hypothyroidism if not followed up carefully. How this can happen is also explained in Chapter Five.

This mixture of different thyroid problems in the same person means that if you bought this book to look up your specific problem, whether hyper- or hypo-, you may benefit from reading the sections on other problems. You may need to know about them, too.

## The Older Woman with 'Hypothermia'

Belle was 73, a widow who lived on her own in the terraced house she had shared for nearly 50 years with her husband. He had died a year before, and she had become a bit reclusive. Her neighbours, who were kindly people, thought it was just part of the process of grieving, but they still looked in on her a few days every week, to keep contact.

Recently, though, Belle had got a bit grumpy. She had put on a lot of weight, lost most of her hair, and seemed a lot slower than she used to be, physically and intellectually. Her neighbour, who was about the same age, became worried when Belle started wearing extra clothing during the day, sitting in her overcoat even on reasonably warm days in the autumn.

Luckily, the neighbour mentioned this to the local district nurse. The nurse realized that, as winter was drawing on, Belle was a prime candidate for hypothermia. So Belle's general practitioner was alerted, and he and the nurse made a joint visit. They found Belle sitting in a cool back room, wearing woolly jumpers and an overcoat. She was a little confused, sleepy, and wondering why anyone should call in the doctor and nurse on her behalf. They explained her neighbour's concern, and gently took her pulse. It was 58 beats per minute. Her temperature under the tongue was low, too, at 36.5 degrees centigrade.

The nurse made her a cup of hot sweet tea, and the doctor took some blood from her. They called her daughter, who lived not far away, and she made sure Belle was looked after for a few days. The blood test showed very low thyroxine levels, and high thyroid-stimulating hormone (TSH) levels. Belle was diagnosed with hypothyroidism due to failure of the thyroid to respond to TSH.

Only a day or two after being prescribed thyroxine, Belle was back to her old lively self. A year on she has lost her excess weight and looks far better. Her hair is growing back, and she looks ten years younger. She goes out with her friends and is often the life and soul of the group.

### The Young Mother Who Was 'Tired All the Time'

Not all cases of extreme hypothyroidism (also known as myxoedema) are as obvious as Belle's. Hypothyroid states can be missed as easily as hyperthyroid ones, even in doctors.

For Dr Brown, going back to work after having her baby was the hardest thing she had ever done. She worried all the time about leaving him. Unsurprisingly he cried every morning as his mother dropped him at the nursery: it took time for his mother to recover from the 'drenching panic' on her journey to work. A year later she found herself losing her hair. She blamed the hairdresser, and did not think for a moment she had myxoedema.

Life remained a struggle. Her finances improved, so she was able to work less. She felt that having a baby had 'dented her brain'. She became a regular at her own doctor's surgery for a series of minor complaints. Her inability to cope, her ebbing confidence, her increasing bulk and her 'mad-professor' hair all became part of her.

She became very slow in making decisions. Her family and friends knew all about her struggles with her household and being a parent, her sleeping during the day and her early nights.

She had a second child two years later. By the time he was two, it dawned on Dr Brown that she needed help. Now, any job, from getting dressed to seeing a patient, was a mountain to climb. She finally described to her doctor what 'tired all the time' meant for her, and asked if her thyroid function could be tested. She had very low thyroid-stimulating hormone (TSH) and thyroxine levels. She was severely hypothyroid because of the failure of her pituitary gland to produce TSH.

Now Dr Brown checks the thyroid function of all mothers with postnatal depression or who are overly concerned about their baby. Her spell of tiredness has led her to investigate all her 'tired all the time' patients. She wants to identify those with low thyroid function before they become severely myxoedemic. She says that thyroxine is giving her back her energy. Her surgeries are enjoyable again, housework is achievable and potty training possible. She says that her challenge is how she can repay her older child, now seven years old, for growing up with a permanently exhausted mother.

Dr Brown has said it all. Thyroid disease, if undiagnosed, can destroy the quality of life in so many ways. Diagnosed and treated, it is no more than a bad memory and a temporary inconvenience.

An underactive thyroid (hypothyroidism) is the most common of all thyroid problems. By far the most cases are due to a problem in the thyroid itself: in this condition, defined as 'primary hypothyroidism', it simply 'gives up' on thyroid hormone production. This was Belle's condition. Fewer cases are due, like Dr Brown's, to the pituitary gland failing to deliver TSH to the thyroid (see Chapter One). This is defined as 'secondary hypothyroidism'.


## Hypothyroidism and Myxoedema

Here we must differentiate between hypothyroidism and 'myxoedema'. Hypothyroidism describes the state of low thyroid activity, regardless of whether or not the person with it shows the whole range of symptoms that come with it. Myxoedema is an extreme form of hypothyroidism, with the thickening and firm swelling of the skin of the face and limbs that makes people with it look so different from their old selves. People with myxoedema have hypothyroidism, but not all people with hypothyroidism have myxoedema.

The first description of myxoedema in an adult (the changes were already recognized in what were then known as 'cretinous' children) was by Dr W W Gill in 1874. He entitled his paper 'On a cretinoid state supervening in adult life in women'.[1] His description holds good today:

> The skin of the face and particularly of the eyelids, becoming thick, semi-transparent and waxy. The face was generally pale, but had a delicate blush on the cheeks. The eyelids were swollen and ridged, and hang down flaccidly on the cheeks. They did not pit on being squeezed. The skin was singularly dry. It was harsh and rough to the touch: the hairs were feebly developed, and no trace of fatty secretion could be found. Within two years the complexion was pale yellow.

In today's words, over 80 per cent of people with primary hypothyroidism (due to thyroid problems) have skin that is rough, dry and covered with fine scales. Only around 10 per cent of people with secondary hypothyroidism (due to pituitary problems) show these skin changes: instead their predominant change is wrinkles.

## Common Causes of an Underactive Thyroid

In most people with an underactive thyroid, the thyroid gland has lost most of its ability to produce the thyroid hormones T3 and T4. The most common cause of this is an auto-immune disorder, known to doctors as Hashimoto's disease (see below). If you've read Chapter Three this may surprise you, because it was explained there that Graves' disease, which is a severe form of hyperthyroidism, is also an auto-immune disorder. So how can a similar mechanism produce such dissimilar diseases?

Put simply, in Graves' disease, the abnormal auto-immune antibody, when it attaches itself to the thyroid cells, stimulates them to over-produce the thyroid hormones T3 and T4. It does not destroy the cells. In the Hashimoto type of auto-immune hypothyroidism, on the other hand, the reaction between the auto-immune antibody and the cells causes inflammation and destruction, destroying the cells' ability to produce thyroid hormones, and leaving the gland as a mass of scar tissue, eventually producing little or even no thyroid hormone. The second most common cause of hypothyroidism in adults is the treatment of hyperthyroidism! Many hyperthyroid people, who have had to have surgery to remove most of their thyroid glands (usually about seven-eighths of the gland is removed), become hypothyroid afterwards. This is not a real problem, because the symptoms are easily reversed by giving the appropriate amount of thyroid hormone (usually thyroxine) every day to compensate for the loss. But it must be recognized and treated, so everyone who has had thyroid surgery or radio-iodine therapy is asked for regular checks of thyroid function, to ensure that they are not falling into the underactive (hypothyroid) range.

Silent thyroiditis and subacute thyroiditis, already described in Chapter Three, can also cause hypothyroidism, usually following a brief period of hyperthyroid activity. Happily, these two forms of thyroiditis are usually temporary, the person returning to normal health after three or four months. Occasionally the thyroid damage is irreversible, and the resultant hypothyroidism needs lifelong treatment.

## Rarer Causes of Hypothyroidism

There are other, much rarer causes of hypothyroidism, listed here for completeness. They include diseases of the skin and connective tissues, known as amyloidosis and scleroderma, which invade the thyroid tissue, causing scarring. People with these diseases have other evidence of the illnesses, such as chronic lung disease (in the case of amyloidosis) or tightening of the skin of the face and in the throat and oesophagus (in scleroderma). As an underactive thyroid is a recognized complication of these illnesses, patients are usually tested for it at routine follow-ups for their primary illness.

Both iodine deficiency and iodine excess can cause hypothyroidism. In iodine deficiency this is easily explained: thyroid hormones contain molecules of iodine at their heart (see Chapter Two), and without enough iodine, not enough thyroid hormone can be secreted into the circulation.

Iodine excess is a little more complex. Today, there are few areas where the iodine levels in the water and food are excessive, but some people over-do their intake of iodine, as a so-called health supplement, in the mistaken belief that it is doing them good. In fact the extra iodine in the circulation shuts down the thyroid gland's production of thyroid hormone, giving exactly the opposite of the desired effect. As iodine passes through the placenta from mother into the developing fetus, this can be particularly harmful in pregnancy. The babies of such pregnancies can be born with goitres and low thyroid activity – and this can cause severe brain damage if not treated soon after birth. Mothers-to-be who give themselves extra vitamins and minerals should take professional advice about them, and not self-treat.

## The Symptoms of Hypothyroidism

People with hypothyroidism share the same galaxy of symptoms, regardless of the cause. It affects both sexes and all ages. It can be mild, with only a few pointers to the illness, or very severe, even producing coma and death. The table below lists the symptoms, but many people only show a few of them. Hypothyroidism should be suspected in any adult whose mental and physical characteristics have recently changed, so that they are showing several of the following symptoms and signs for the first time. Hypothyroidism, particularly of the Hashimoto type, comes on very slowly, so that the changes can be subtle and gradual. To begin with only a minority of features may be present. Sometimes the change is so slow that even closest family members do not notice it. Often it takes an occasional visitor to remark upon the change in someone whom they have not seen for a year or two for the penny to drop, and action to be taken.

# The Features of Hypothyroidism

| Symptoms | Signs |
|---|---|
| Feeling physically tired all the time | Slow movements |
| Lethargy/lassitude/laziness | Slow speech |
| Sleepiness at inappropriate times | Hoarse speech |
| Mental dullness | Slow pulse |
| Depression | Dry skin |
| Intolerance to cold | Thickened, swollen skin of the face and limbs (myxoedema) |
| Weight gain | Lack of sweat |
| Loss of appetite | Less active reflexes |
| Constipation | Slower reflexes |
| Menstrual problems | With or without goitre |
| Joint pains | Abnormal sensations – pins and needles and numbness |

Happily, for the vast majority of people with hypothyroidism, once the diagnosis is made and the treatment started, all the symptoms and signs listed above can be quickly reversed – because they are all linked to the lack of thyroid hormone activity in the body. And thyroid hormone is very easy to replace.

Professor Hashimoto was a Japanese physician who as long ago as 1912 reported on a series of people with goitres in which microscopic examination showed evidence of long-standing inflammation.[2] The condition has been called Hashimoto's disease ever since.

It used to be thought that Hashimoto's disease was rare: in fact the diagnosis was usually only made after examining a goitre removed at operation. Now, however, we know that such chronic thyroid inflammation has many guises, leading sometimes to goitre and sometimes to loss of thyroid tissue (in medical terms, atrophy), so that it can occur without any thyroid swelling.

The underlying mechanism in all these cases (lumped together as 'Hashimoto's thyroiditis') is auto-immunity, as described above. Somehow the body turns against its own thyroid tissue, and gradually destroys it. The experts divide cases according to their appearance under the microscope. There are 'fibrous' cases in which the appearance is just of massive scarring – fibrosis. There are 'lymphocytic' cases in which the thyroid is a mass of lymphocytes – specific white blood cells associated with immune reactions. This is the usual case in hypothyroidism occurring for the first time in childhood, adolescence and young adulthood. A temporary form of this type of thyroiditis occurs in women just after giving birth: this is 'postpartum thyroiditis', which usually disappears over a few months.

The consensus seems to have settled towards the use of 'auto-immune thyroiditis' to include all these forms of hypothyroidism. Hashimoto's disease is thus the 'sub-diagnosis' in people with obviously enlarged thyroid glands (goitres), while atrophic thyroiditis is diagnosed in those whose thyroid glands are not visible or palpable.

Whatever the type, auto-immune thyroiditis seems to be on the increase. Some researchers have blamed the increase on the much higher intake of iodine generally in the last few decades, but this is unproven. Whether or not this is the cause, it does seem very common. When Dr B R Hawkins and his colleagues looked for thyroid antibodies (evidence of thyroiditis) in a healthy population chosen at random, they found that around 4 per cent had some thyroid abnormality secondary to auto-immune thyroiditis.[3] And post-mortem tests in elderly women have revealed that 15 per cent of them have thyroid auto-antibodies, though some of these women had not had their illness diagnosed in life.

Why should so many people have problems in their thyroid glands? The answer lies at least partly in their genes. People with Graves' disease (auto-immunity that causes hyperthyroidism) and Hashimoto's disease (auto-immunity that causes hypothyroidism) share closely related genetic make-ups. The technical term is that they share similar 'histocompatibility lymphocyte antigens' (HLA). HLA type determines the details of how our immune systems react to foreign (and our own) proteins.

We know, for example, that people with Graves' disease and people with atrophic thyroiditis tend to produce the HLA-DR3 antigens.[4] There are families with cases of both Graves' disease and Hashimoto's disease: the patients with these two contrasting diseases share the same HLA types. There have even been identical twins, one with Graves' disease and the other with Hashimoto's thyroiditis.[5] And in such families, apparently unaffected relatives show some evidence of thyroid abnormalities which are not enough to cause symptoms.

So hyperthyroidism (Graves' disease) and hypothyroidism (auto-immune thyroiditis, Hashimoto's disease) are not opposite ends of thyroid disease, but are probably two forms of the same illness, with just subtle differences between them.

The proof of this is that some cases of Graves' disease eventually become Hashimoto's disease, with underactivity of the thyroid – and, more rarely, some cases of Hashimoto's disease can turn into Graves' disease.

There are differences between the two, however. Thyroid-stimulating antibody (TSAb – see page 38) is present in Graves' disease but is usually absent in Hashimoto's. The eye symptoms (see Chapter Three) are common in Graves' disease, but usually absent in Hashimoto's. They, differ, too, in the presence of other conditions often associated with thyroid disease.

## Other Auto-immune Diseases Linked to Auto-immune Thyroiditis

Unfortunately, a few people with one auto-immune disorder, such as Graves' or Hashimoto's disease, have others along with it. People with either of these two thyroid diseases are more likely than normal to develop 'Type 1' diabetes, the form of diabetes for which insulin injections are needed. They may also have Addison's disease, in which the cells in the adrenal glands (they lie just above the kidneys) are affected. The adrenal glands normally produce cortisone, and lack of it in Addison's disease causes weakness, loss of energy, low blood pressure and a deep tanning of the skin. As the symptoms of hypothyroidism and Addison's disease obviously overlap, it is usual for doctors to order an endocrine 'screen' to measure cortisone levels as well as thyroid hormone levels in suspected cases.

Much more rarely, the ovaries, parathyroid glands and the pituitary can also be affected by auto-immune problems, in a condition labelled 'polyendocrine auto-immune disease'. This leads, as might be expected, to a host of other symptoms. Ovarian involvement can lead to loss of the menstrual cycle and sterility. The four parathyroid glands (they are like four small peas sitting just behind the thyroid gland) regulate the amount of calcium in the bones. In polyendocrine auto-immune disease, hypo-parathyroidism (underactivity) can lead to loss of calcium and subsequent softening and collapse of the weight-bearing bones. The pituitary regulates the output of hormones from the ovaries/testes, the adrenals, the thyroid and parathyroids, so that its failure produces a host of other symptoms. Happily, once recognized, the missing hormones can soon be replaced.

However, it is not just the other endocrine organs that may be attacked along with the thyroid in auto-immune thyroiditis. People with either Graves' disease or hypothyroidism due to auto-immune problems are also at higher-than-normal risk of auto-immune diseases affecting other parts of the body. Illnesses definitely linked to auto-immune thyroid disease (found more often in people with thyroid disease than in the general population), include:

- pernicious anaemia (in which the anaemia is caused by the body's inability to take up vitamin B12 from food)
- vitiligo (in which the skin pigment becomes very patchy, so that people appear almost 'piebald')
- Sjogren's syndrome (in which the body fluids dry up, leaving the eyes, nose, mouth and throat uncomfortably dry)
- alopecia (bald patches or even complete loss of all hair)

- myasthenia gravis (in which the muscles become much weaker than normal after the slightest exertion)
- chronic hepatitis (persistent liver inflammation)
- thrombocytopenia (in which the lack of platelets in the blood leads to excessive bruising).

Other illnesses that have been proposed as linked to thyroiditis, but for which there is as yet no definite evidence that they are more common in cases of hyperthyroidism or hypothyroidism, include:

- rheumatoid arthritis
- progressive systemic sclerosis (in which there is a general fibrosis, or scarring, in many organs)
- some rare forms of dermatitis
- systemic lupus erythematosus (in which the skin and often the kidneys suffer chronic inflammation)
- polymyalgia rheumatica-giant cell arteritis syndrome. This produces severe muscle pains along with excruciating pain in the temple which can lead to sudden blindness if the sufferer is not treated as an emergency with high doses of steroids.

Don't let this list of illnesses linked to thyroiditis alarm you. It is there because a small number of readers will recognize their own combination of problems among them. If you are one of them, be reassured that modern treatments can help ease both sets of problems, and that they will not clash. You may need a combination of thyroid hormone (usually thyroxine) or anti-thyroid drugs for the thyroid disease plus steroids or other immune-suppressant drugs, including newer drugs such as methotrexate, for the second auto-immune problem. See Chapter Six for more details on treatments.

However, steroids or immune suppressants are not the only possible treatment for hypothyroidism alone: it can always be treated satisfactorily with thyroxine (T4) or tri-iodothyronine (T3).

## Other Forms of Hypothyroidism

Although most cases of hypothyroidism fall into the category of auto-immune disease (see above) there are others with different causes that follow different courses. Two that have already been mentioned (see Chapter Three) are subacute and silent thyroiditis. A third is 'postpartum' hypothyroidism, that is a variant of silent thyroiditis peculiar to the period just after giving birth (hence the word postpartum – the medical term for the period just after a delivery).

All three of these illnesses initially cause hyperthyroidism (overactivity of the thyroid), but may, after two to three weeks, subside into hypothyroidism, a state that lasts for up to three months or a little more, before the person returns to normal. In these cases the hypothyroidism is usually mild, and no treatment except reassurance and good follow-up is needed.

## Postpartum Thyroiditis
Postpartum thyroiditis differs from the other two in that the patient is more likely to show anti-thyroid antibodies in her blood, has a greater risk of the hypothyroidism becoming permanent, and is more likely to have a recurrence of the illness. In one study, 39 per cent of patients with postpartum thyroiditis were still hypothyroid nine months after the illness started, compared with only 17 per cent with non-pregnancy-related silent thyroiditis.[6] In another, 23 per cent of women who had postpartum thyroiditis were still hypothyroid between two and four years after the birth.[7]

## 'Riedel's Thyroiditis'
A fairly rare form of hypothyroidism is 'Riedel's thyroiditis', or 'invasive fibrous thyroiditis', first described by the German Professor Riedel in the 1880s. It mainly affects middle-aged women who complain of pressure in the front of the neck, difficulty in swallowing and breathlessness – as if they are being strangled. Their main problem is the replacement of the thyroxine-producing cells in the thyroid by a dense scar tissue, the technical name for which is fibrosis. Patients with Riedel's thyroiditis have a very hard, swollen thyroid – the texture is like wood or even stone, and it seems stuck to the surrounding tissues in the neck. In contrast, most other goitres (for example those due to Hashimoto's disease) are much softer, and very mobile, so that the skin and muscles can be moved smoothly over and behind them.

Riedel's thyroid disease may be only a part of an illness with fibrosis in other sites, such as inside the abdomen, or behind the eyes, or in the liver and lungs. If you are diagnosed as having Riedel's thyroiditis, you may need special scans to rule out this form of general scarring. Up to half of all people with a Riedel's thyroid become hypothyroid. Unlike other forms of hypothyroidism, which often recover spontaneously, Riedel's hypothyroidism is permanent, and needs lifelong treatment.

Hypothyroidism can also be a secondary effect of other diseases. One, for example, is haemochromatosis, an inherited condition in which the body cannot deal with iron efficiently. Deposits of excess iron in the thyroid sometimes lead to hypothyroidism in such patients, leading to a fibrous reaction not unlike (though not as severe as) Riedel's disease.

## Post-radiation and Post-operative Hypothyroidism

The most common form of hypothyroidism that is not auto-immune is post-radiation or post-operative hypothyroidism. This is hypothyroidism brought on by treatment either for problems in the neck and nearby tissues, or by treatment for hyperthyroidism.

People with lymphomas (tumours of the lymph glands) often have to have their necks irradiated to destroy the affected glands. Many studies in such patients have established that between a quarter and half of them then become hypothyroid. It usually takes from two to seven years after the radiotherapy before the low thyroid state is recognized, although it may start within a year. Radiotherapy to the mouth and throat for cancer can also lead to hypothyroidism, as can spinal radiation for leukaemias and tumours of the brain and spinal cord.

It is important to know about this, because people often blame their tiredness and low state on their original illness, and fear that it may be coming back, when all they need is a thyroid test. As with treatment of all forms of hypothyroidism, the patient usually feels dramatically better within a day or two, and the improvement in general health is sustained.

A form of radiation therapy that commonly leads to hypothyroidism is radio-iodine treatment (see Chapter Five). This is given for hyperthyroidism, particularly for Graves' disease (see Chapter Three), when there is an urgent need to damp down excessive thyroid activity. In Chapter One it was explained that iodine given by mouth is very specifically taken up by the thyroid gland. Radioactive iodine acts just like normal iodine, in that it is taken up almost exclusively by the thyroid, where it destroys most of the thyroxine-producing cells.

Radio-iodine treatment (the iodine isotope used is $I^{131}$) has dramatic results. The patient quickly returns to normal. However, it is often difficult to judge exactly the right dose for each patient, so that in some people too much thyroid tissue is destroyed. This leaves them hypothyroid. When high doses are given, around half of all patients are hypothyroid a year later: ten years later this figure rises to 70 per cent.[8] With lower doses the corresponding figures are 12 and 33 per cent respectively.[9]

Some experts suggest that if people who have had radio-iodine treatment are followed up for long enough, all of them would be found to have become hypothyroid eventually. That may be an extreme view, but it does mean that everyone who has had this treatment for hyperthyroidism should be followed up regularly for the rest of their lives, to make sure that they are not slowly becoming hypothyroid. The process is a slow one, so that the changes and symptoms may not be obvious, and could even be blamed on old age. Blood levels of TSH, T4 and T3 will soon make the diagnosis clear, and the proper thyroid hormone replacement treatment will be started. This treatment should dramatically improve things.

Surgery is another treatment for hyperthyroidism that can lead to a hypothyroid state. Different studies over the last 40 years have claimed that between 3 and 70 per cent of patients become hypothyroid after surgery for Graves' disease. Even with today's sophisticated surgery, the hypothyroidism rate after such operations is still probably between 10 and 30 per cent.

Whether you become hypothyroid after surgery depends largely on how much thyroid tissue the surgeon leaves behind, but there is no hard and fast rule. Some people who are left with a fairly substantial amount of thyroid tissue become hypothyroid, and others, left with only a tiny remnant, can become hyperthyroid (thyrotoxic) again, as the remaining cells hugely over-produce the hormone thyroxine.

It's difficult to predict who will become hypothyroid after surgery. Some studies suggest the risk is higher in older people, some say younger adults are at highest risk; yet others find that age makes no difference. It does seem more likely when the person lives in an area with low natural iodine levels in the water and food.

Most people who become hypothyroid after surgery do so within a year. About 20 per cent of all people undergoing thyroid surgery for

Graves' disease become hypothyroid around three months after the surgery, but by the sixth month their thyroid becomes normal again. So every person undergoing thyroid surgery is watched closely for the first year, and treatment only started if their hypothyroidism is severe or shows no signs of improving.

People who have thyroid surgery to remove single nodules or who have part of a goitre removed for cosmetic reasons, rather than hyperthyroidism, do not become permanently hypothyroid after surgery, although they may be a little hypothyroid for a few weeks. Their remaining thyroid tissue will provide enough thyroid hormone to keep them normal.


### Drug-induced Hypothyroidism

As well as radio-iodine and surgery, an overactive thyroid (hyperthyroidism) can be treated with drugs that prevent the thyroid gland from producing the thyroid hormones T3 and T4. These are described in Chapter Five, in the treatment of hyperthyroidism. The dose is usually carefully chosen so that they leave the person taking them in a 'euthyroid' (normal thyroid) state.

However, some drugs prescribed for other illnesses may have an anti-thyroid action, so that they can cause people with normal thyroid glands to become hypothyroid. The best known of these is lithium, a drug used mainly for 'bipolar disorder', a condition in which people have swings of mood between depression and unreasonable elation (or 'mania'). It's difficult to understand why lithium affects thyroid function. Higher-than-usual anti-thyroid antibody levels have been reported in some people taking lithium who become hypothyroid, suggesting that they had previous thyroid disease before taking the drug. But others become hypothyroid even though they showed no evidence of previous thyroid disease.

Whatever the cause, 15 per cent of people taking lithium for between two and nine years (an average of five years) have hypothyroid symptoms, with high TSH and low T4 levels.[10] If you have been diagnosed as hypothyroid and have been taking lithium, it is very likely that your thyroid problem is a side-effect of your therapy.

The same statement can be made of the drug amiodarone (see Chapter Two). This is a highly successful drug for easing and preventing angina (pain due to poor circulation to the heart muscle) and correcting abnormal heart rhythms (it is an 'anti-arrhythmic' agent). However, in almost everyone taking amiodarone there are subtle changes in the thyroid, usually only picked up on laboratory tests.

In a minority of people taking amiodarone, these changes lead to symptoms. Some become hyperthyroid (see Chapter Three); others become hypothyroid. The hypothyroid symptoms usually begin within a year of starting to take amiodarone, but can occasionally start later. There have even been very rare reports of people dying from coma due to profound hypothyroidism with myxoedema.[11]

Amiodarone remains in the body for months, so if your hypothyroidism has been caused by it the hypothyroidism may persist and need to be treated long after the amiodarone is stopped. The treatment has to be conducted with special care, because most people on amiodarone have heart problems, and giving them thyroid hormone such as T4 may make these heart problems worse. It is a question of balancing the benefit of improving the hypothyroid state with doing one's best to avoid making the heart worse. Needless to say, people on long-term amiodarone should have regular checks of their thyroid function (blood TSH, T4 and T3 levels).

People with epilepsy are another group who may need regular checks on whether they are becoming hypothyroid. Two drugs to control epileptic seizures ('anticonvulsants'), carbamazepine and phenytoin, reduce blood levels of T4, probably because they speed up its breakdown by the liver. However, although people taking these drugs have relatively low thyroxine levels, it is rare for levels to be so low as to cause symptoms of hypothyroidism. The problem comes when people with epilepsy are asked to take both their anticonvulsant and another drug likely to cause hypothyroidism, such as lithium. Then they may need to be given thyroxine as well, or to change their anticonvulsant to one that does not affect the thyroid, such as valproate. People who have both hypothyroidism and epilepsy (not an uncommon combination of illnesses) may have to take larger-than-usual doses of thyroxine to avoid hypothyroid symptoms.

Other drugs which lower T4 levels include sulphonamides (antibacterial agents sometimes still used for urine infections), sulphonylureas (used in adult-onset diabetes to lower blood glucose levels), and ethionamide (a treatment for advanced breast and prostate cancer). They, like anticonvulsants, rarely cause obvious hypothyroidism, but when they are prescribed to people already on treatment for hypothyroidism, the thyroxine dose may need to be raised.


## Central Hypothyroidism

In 'central hypothyroidism' the flaw is not in the thyroid gland itself, but in its control by the pituitary (see Chapter One). Put simply, the pituitary gland is not sending its thyroid-stimulating hormone (TSH) message to the thyroid to release T4 and T3.

The most common cause of central hypothyroidism is 'pituitary adenoma', a benign tumour in the pituitary which compresses the normal, TSH-secreting, part of the pituitary gland. With less TSH in the circulation, the thyroid produces less T4 and T3, and the patient becomes hypothyroid. This is starkly different from the other type of pituitary tumour described in Chapter Three, which actively secretes TSH and causes hyperthyroidism.

There are a few reports of other tumours around and in the pituitary that can cause hypothyroidism, but they are very rare, and beyond the scope of this book. One, for example, is 'craniopharyngioma', a tumour which arises in the floor of the skull just under the brain, and is more common in younger than older adults. It is enough to state here that if the thyroid tests suggest a pituitary cause for hypothyroidism (for example lower-than-usual blood levels of TSH, T4 and T3), then the next steps are to look for a cause in the pituitary or craniopharyngeal area. This starts with an X-ray of the skull, and may be followed up by brain scans.

Very rarely, severe blood loss, as after an accident or after a difficult birth, leads to the 'death' or 'infarction' of the pituitary cells due to lack of blood flow to them. The pituitary is particularly vulnerable to such 'shock'. It used to be so common after severe bleeding during and after childbirth that it was even given a name, 'Sheehan's syndrome', after the doctor who first described it.[12]

With the whole pituitary gone, women with Sheehan's syndrome (or men who have the equivalent after severe blood loss) have more than hypothyroidism. They are also deficient in the other hormones whose outputs are normally controlled by the pituitary. So while they have the usual problems of hypothyroidism, such as hating the cold, being constipated and always being tired, lethargic and mentally dull, they also:

- are unable to turn on a defence against infection (due to their inability to produce cortisone)
- in men, become impotent, with no sexual urges and shrinking testicles (because of the lack of male sex hormones)
- in women, lose their periods, become infertile, and have shrinking breasts (because of the loss of female sex hormones)
- in either sex, lose their pubic and armpit hair
- become weak, develop low blood pressure when standing up, and lose pigment in their nipples (because they lose the ability to produce adrenaline).

Sheehan's syndrome comes on only a few weeks after the birth. Because of the host of symptoms, and because it is easily linked with the difficult childbirth, it should not be difficult to diagnose. The treatment, of course, has to be directed to replacing all the defects – the sex hormones, the cortisone, adrenaline and thyroid hormone. This treatment will be needed for the rest of the woman's life.

Happily, Sheehan's syndrome is much rarer than it used to be in developed countries, where the risks of not quickly replacing blood loss during and after childbirth are now very well known. But it is still a major cause of severe illness and even death in the developing world, where childbirth can still be very traumatic and dangerous for the mother, and safe and adequate blood transfusion is still often just a dream.

Something akin to Sheehan's syndrome may occur in people, men and women alike, who have lost a lot of blood in accidents, or who have had small blood clots in, or bleeds from, defective blood vessels in the area of the pituitary or hypothalamus. Very occasionally it can happen to people who need to have radiotherapy to the brain for tumours arising close to the pituitary. The underlying mechanism is the same as that for Sheehan's syndrome – loss of the pituitary cells which produce TSH.

Whatever the cause of the central hypothyroidism, the treatment is first to restore normal thyroid function, so people with it are given thyroxine in just the same way as people with hypothyroidism due to the more usual causes. However, as many people with central hypothyroidism are also lacking in other hormones, such as cortisone and sex hormones, these other hormones must form part of the treatment, too.

If the cause is a pituitary tumour this has also to be tackled, so that simply giving thyroxine in every case of hypothyroidism is a mistake. The cause of the low thyroid function must be found in every case before treatment can be started. Although only four cases of hypothyroidism in every hundred have pituitary problems as their cause, that cause must be found if they are to be treated properly and correctly.

# Part Three
# Treatment

# Chapter Five

# Treating an Overactive Thyroid Thyrotoxicosis

Around 60 per cent of all cases of hyperthyroidism take the form of 'thyrotoxicosis'. Strictly speaking, thyrotoxicosis is the name for the illness caused by hyperthyroidism. It can also be called Graves' Disease.

In medicine, the ideal treatment is always to find the cause of an illness and eliminate it. In most people with thyrotoxicosis, however, this isn't possible. We just don't know exactly why the thyroid glands produce the excessive amounts of thyroid hormone that are causing the symptoms. For the few people with pituitary thyrotoxicosis (see page 42), removing the pituitary tumour is the answer. Similarly, for those whose thyrotoxicosis is due to over-treatment with thyroid hormone (see page 109), the obvious treatment is simply to adjust the dose of the hormone.

For the vast majority of people with thyrotoxicosis, however, the only strategy is to destroy most of the overactive thyroid gland, so that much less thyroid hormone (T4 and T3) is produced. This leaves the doctors with one of three choices:

1. giving 'anti-thyroid' drugs
2. giving radiotherapy (i.e. asking the patient to swallow a dose of 'radio-iodine') to destroy the gland
3. removing most of the gland with surgery

Unfortunately, making this choice is not simple, and there are no hard-and-fast rules about which person should have which treatment. Opinions differ among thyroid specialists about which type of treatment is suitable for which type of patient. The final decision depends partly on the patients' characteristics (such as age), and on the doctor's own experience. More and more, the decision is up to the patients themselves. So the three main types of treatment – drugs, surgery or radiotherapy – are described in the following pages to help you, if you are needing treatment, to make up your own mind.

Anti-thyroid drugs have been the mainstay of treatment for thyrotoxicosis since the 1940s, so that their advantages and drawbacks are very well known.[1] They block the ability of the thyroid gland to make T4 and T3, so that blood levels of these hormones fall, and the symptoms disappear accordingly.

The two types of drug used today are the thiouracils and the imidazoles. Today, the only thiouracil still in use is propylthiouracil, or PTU. Of the imidazoles, the one used in North America is methimazole, and that used in Europe is carbimazole. As carbimazole rapidly turns into methimazole in the body, the two drugs are interchangeable.

Both PTU and methimazole/carbimazole are very effective in controlling thyrotoxicosis due to Graves' disease, so that the choice between them often comes down to the preference of the prescribing doctor. PTU comes in 50-mg tablets, and methimazole in 5- or 20-mg tablets, the difference reflecting the fact that methimazole is a more potent drug, weight for weight.

The starting dose for PTU is usually 100 mg three times daily, coming down to a daily dose of 50 to 100 mg as the person improves. The corresponding starting dose of methimazole/carbimazole is 20 to 30 mg daily, falling to 2.5 or 5 mg once a day or even on each alternate day, after the symptoms have receded.

How fast you recover after starting either type of drug depends on how overactive the thyroid is initially, how much hormone is already stored in the gland (the bigger the goitre, the longer the recovery may take), and how much, and how often, the drug is given. Many doctors now prefer methimazole/carbimazole to PTU because the former's once-a-day dose gives more reliable results (and people find it easier to take a once-a-day tablet). Recovery to a normal thyroid state seems faster on methimazole/carbimazole, and the lower doses of methimazole/carbimazole may be safer.

Most of the side-effects of the anti-thyroid drugs are 'allergic' in type. They include rashes, urticaria (swollen red lumps like nettle rash), fever and joint pains. They are reported in from 1 to 5 per cent of people taking them,[2] the higher figure being linked to the higher doses. They are usually temporary, the rash fading again within a week on treatment with an antihistamine tablet, without the need to stop the anti-thyroid drug.

Serious side-effects are very much less frequent (around two to five people per thousand given either drug). They include anaemias, 'agranulocytosis' (loss of certain white blood cells), hepatitis (inflammation of the liver), joint pains and inflammation of the blood vessels ('vasculitis'). Apart from agranulocytosis, which seems to be divided equally between the two drugs, and is the most serious of them all, these side-effects are all more common in those on PTU than on methimazole/carbimazole.

Side-effects are much more likely to arise in the first three months of treatment, but they can start later, and occasionally more than a year later. Although agranulocytosis usually occurs very suddenly, so that regular white blood cell counts may not pick it up early, people on these drugs are usually asked to give regular blood samples to check on their red and white blood cells. However, this system is not foolproof, so that people given anti-thyroid drugs are asked particularly to report to their doctors any symptom that might raise suspicions of agranulocytosis. This is because the granulocytes are the white blood cells that are the body's first line of protection against germs: without them people die within days of overwhelming infections. The main initial symptoms of agranulocytosis are a high fever and a very sore, raw throat. If this happens to you when on an anti-thyroid drug, you must see your doctor at once.

Caught early, agranulocytosis begins to recede soon after stopping the treatment and starting the patient on a powerful antibiotic. The white blood cell count is back to normal within 14 days. People who develop agranulocytosis on an anti-thyroid drug are usually still thyrotoxic. They cannot be transferred on to another anti-thyroid drug. Instead they may be given iodine, a beta-blocker or lithium, until they can be given radio-iodine or surgery.

### The Results with Anti-thyroid Drugs
The main aim of anti-thyroid drugs is to return thyroid hormone levels, and therefore the person, to a normal thyroid state. Most experts recommend taking them for between one and two years before stopping them, though there is good evidence that even longer courses are better, especially in children.[3] The longer the course, the more likely it is that the person will remain with a normal thyroid state after the drug is stopped.

In most adults, if the thyrotoxic symptoms return after the person has had two long courses of the drugs, then they are advised to have either surgery or radio-iodine treatment. However, some people prefer to continue to take a small dose of methimazole/carbimazole for many years, rather than undergo surgery or radiotherapy. As the drugs are relatively safe there are no strong objections to this, provided that the person undergoes regular blood checks.

It is very difficult to predict, at the start of the treatment, who will respond with a 'remission' (no return of the thyrotoxicosis after stopping treatment) and who will not. As the thyrotoxic state diminishes, with the heart rate slowing and the person feeling much better, regular visits to the doctor are needed to check on thyroid function. These are the simple blood tests for TSH, T4 and T3 described in Chapter One. This has two aims – to make sure that the person is no longer thyrotoxic, and to make sure, too, that she has not slid into hypothyroidism (underactivity of the thyroid).

At each doctor visit, the thyroid gland will be checked to make sure that it is not enlarging – an indication, usually, of hypothyroidism developing, and less often of continuing thyrotoxic disease. As the treatment continues, pointers that the person is entering a remission include a decreasing goitre, the ability to cut down on drug dose without the return of symptoms, and subtle changes in the ratio between T3 and T4 levels in the blood. The doctor may also measure thyroid antibody (TSAb) levels, which fall as a remission begins. If the TSAb level remains high during anti-thyroid drug treatment, this suggests that the thyrotoxicosis will return should it be stopped.

So, people taking anti-thyroid drugs for thyrotoxicosis should find that their thyroid glands become smaller, and that they remain normal on gradually lowering doses of the drug. They can eventually stop the drug with confidence that, should the illness return, it can be spotted early and treated before it causes any obvious ill-health.

If the illness does return, it will probably do so within three to six months after stopping the drug. Sometimes the relapse can be caught before it causes symptoms, because the initial sign is a rise in T3 (but not T4) levels, so the doctor will continue to measure T4 and T3 levels at monthly intervals for a year or more after stopping treatment.

Unfortunately, thyrotoxicosis may recur years after successful treatment. In one study, 91 per cent of patients given anti-thyroid drugs for fewer than two years relapsed into thyrotoxicosis again within five years of stopping their drug.[4] Many experts, therefore, insist that the initial treatment lasts at least two years, and often longer. The longer the initial treatment period, it seems, the less likely the disease will recur later. Relapse into thyrotoxicosis is especially likely in women just after giving birth. Among women who had been given anti-thyroid drugs for thyrotoxicosis, but were in remission during their pregnancies, half developed the disease again in the first few weeks after giving birth.[5]

The fact that so many people have recurrent thyrotoxicosis after what initially seemed a cure of their illness has made it essential that everyone who has had the disease is followed up for life. The basic strategy is simple. If the patient is a child, then recurrences can be treated with a second course of anti-thyroid drugs. In a young adult whose thyrotoxicosis recurs, there is a choice between a second course of an anti-thyroid drug or radio-iodine therapy (see later in this chapter). In older adults with a second bout of thyrotoxicosis, radio-iodine is used, largely because second and further courses of anti-thyroid drugs have proved less successful. In fact, radio-iodine may well be the best choice even for their first bout of illness.

**Other Drugs Used for Hyperthyroidism**
To the specific anti-thyroid drugs mentioned above must be added another group of drugs occasionally used to help treat thyrotoxicosis. These include iodide, potassium perchlorate, lithium, and beta-blockers.

*Iodide*
Nowadays, iodide is used in three circumstances. It is given to patients just before surgery, to patients in thyrotoxic storm (see page 97), and together with radio-iodine therapy. Iodide stops the release of the stores of already-formed T3 and T4 from the thyroid, so it works fast in emergencies and 'cools down' the overactive thyroid quickly, making it ideal as a preparation for surgery and for thyrotoxic storm. However, the thyroid quickly 'escapes' from this blocking action, so the iodide effect does not last long. Sometimes after it is stopped the thyrotoxicosis worsens. This makes it imperative that

iodide is used only as a stop-gap while a permanent solution to the problem (such as surgery or radio-iodine) is being planned.

Iodide is usually given before surgery, as drops of potassium iodide solution three times a day. In life-threatening emergencies, as in thyrotoxic storm, it is given intravenously, as sodium iodide. When it is given along with radio-iodine treatment, it is usually started one week before giving the radio-iodine. Patients given this combined treatment are followed up closely afterwards because they may suddenly develop hypothyroidism. Why this should happen is not entirely clear.

This treatment has its drawbacks. It may make some people with toxic nodular goitre (see Chapter Three) much worse, a reaction called the Jod-Basedow phenomenon after the nineteenth-century doctor who first described it. And some people react with an acne-like rash, inflamed salivary glands and inflammation of the small blood vessels ('vasculitis').

A development onwards from iodide includes the 'iodinated contrast agents', normally used for X-rays of the gall-bladder. They, like iodide, are used to manage thyrotoxic storm and for very fast control in people needing thyroidectomy (surgery to remove the thyroid). They are given once daily or once every three days just before surgery.

*Potassium Perchlorate*
Potassium perchlorate blocks the transport of iodide inside the thyroid cells, so it used to be used for thyrotoxicosis until better drugs such as carbimazole and PTU, with less toxic effects (the potassium perchlorate caused anaemia and stomach ulcers), were introduced. It is still used in the Jod-Basedow reaction (see above), which does not respond well to the usual anti-thyroid drugs. In doses of 40 to 120 mg per day it does not appear to be toxic.[6]

*Lithium*
Lithium is concentrated, like iodine, in the thyroid gland, and blocks release of thyroid hormone so that it does quieten down an overactive thyroid. However, it offers no advantage over the conventional anti-thyroid drugs, and gives decidedly more severe side-effects than them. Its use is therefore confined to treating thyrotoxic storm in patients who are allergic to iodide.

*Beta-blockers*

Beta-blockers are widely used to ease the symptoms in thyrotoxicosis in many patients, along with other anti-thyroid treatment such as anti-thyroid drugs, radio-iodine and surgery. They have no significant direct effect on the thyroid itself, but they relieve very annoying symptoms such as shakiness, palpitations, anxiety and, often most important to patients, intolerance to heat.

Beta-blockers are hardly ever used alone in the long-term management of thyrotoxicosis, except in those mild cases of thyroiditis (see Chapter Three) that are self-limiting. There are dozens of different beta-blockers; each thyroid specialist has his or her own favourite. Suffice it to state here that they all end with 'olol'! They are usually given as a long-acting once-daily tablet or capsule, although in emergencies they can be given as an intravenous drip.

Common side-effects of beta-blockers include nausea, headache, tiredness, sleeplessness and depression. They may worsen asthma, so are only given to people with chest conditions with caution.

## Radio-iodine

Radio-iodine (radioactive iodine) is by far the most widely used treatment for thyrotoxicosis. Naturally, fears about the dangers of radioactivity (the rise of public opinion against nuclear power is one example) make many people apprehensive about any radiotherapy. These fears are heightened by the fact that thyrotoxicosis is not cancer. Most people accept radiotherapy for cancer, because their lives are under immediate threat. It is different for people with thyrotoxicosis, for which other treatments are available, and which, in most cases, is not a killing disease in itself.

Thankfully, radio-iodine has been around as a treatment for thyroid disease since the mid-1940s, so there has been plenty of time to study in great detail its benefits and risks. It has turned out to be an ideal form of treatment. It can be claimed as highly effective and very safe.

The use of radio-iodine depends on the fact that the thyroid gland takes up any swallowed iodine more than 100 times more than any other tissue in the body. So a small dose of iodine by mouth goes virtually entirely into the thyroid gland. Add radioactivity to the dose, and all that radioactivity therefore centres upon the thyroid.

Radioactivity damages the cells, acting effectively like an internal 'burn', causing the thyroid hormone-producing cells first to become inflamed, and then to die off. Over many years, the gland withers (the medical word is 'atrophies') and becomes scar tissue.

How much thyroid tissue is destroyed by the radio-iodine depends on the dose given and how overactive the gland is in the first place. People with a smaller thyroid need less, people with a large toxic nodular goitre need more. Much depends on how avidly the thyroid takes up iodine (this is measured from a small test dose given a few days before the planned treatment), and whether the person has had an anti-thyroid drug beforehand. If one has been used it is stopped at least three days before the radio-iodine is given.

How much radio-iodine is given is still a matter of debate among the experts. Some try to give a dose that is low enough to leave the thyroid with some ability to produce thyroid hormone, so that the patient has the chance of being euthyroid (with normal thyroid hormone production) afterwards. Others feel that a high enough dose should be given to obliterate all thyroid activity, on the grounds that it is easy to give replacement thyroid hormone therapy afterwards, and that it will ensure that the thyrotoxicosis will not return.

In fact, most people are cured of their thyrotoxicosis by a single dose of radio-iodine, and most eventually become hypothyroid (with an underactive thyroid), so that they need to take thyroid hormone (usually as thyroxine).

Radio-iodine (almost universally given today as the isotope $I^{131}$) has an eight-day 'half life'. That is, its radioactivity declines by half every eight days. So the patient is mildly radioactive for about two weeks. However, the radioactivity (it is called beta-irradiation) has a 'path length' (the distance which the radioactivity spreads) of only 1 to 2 millimetres. This guarantees that the damage is limited to the thyroid gland only, and not to any distant tissues, or to the patient's family and friends. There is no need for anyone to worry about long-term side-effects of being in contact with someone who has just taken radio-iodine. Close relatives of people who have just been given radio-iodine often ask about the possible danger to themselves. Should they be in close proximity to them for a long time, such as on a car journey? Should they sleep together? Are there dangers in making love? Is the problem worse when the person develops a cold or allergy, with sneezing? Does the radio-iodine complicate taking the contraceptive pill? The answer in each case is that radio-iodine does not cause any problems in any of these ways. Life should just go on as before.

Organizing radio-iodine treatment can, however, cause problems for the medical profession's regulatory bodies. For example, if you vomit immediately after swallowing your dose of radio-iodine, this contaminates the area, and it has to be mopped up by experts! Our local biochemist, who is in charge of all radio-iodine treatments, has had to deal with road-side 'spills' after people have stopped to be sick and unwittingly polluted the kerbside. So if you are sick just after taking your dose, you must report it to the doctors in charge.

Radio-iodine is given as a single capsule or a single drink. The radioactivity quickly concentrates in the thyroid gland, which can sometimes be tender for a day or two afterwards. The thyroid symptoms may even get worse for a short time, as some stored thyroid hormone is released from the damaged tissues. Within a week to a month or so, the thyroid then becomes normal.

During this initial period most people are given beta-blocking drugs to control the symptoms (people still have palpitations, a fast heartbeat, feel nervous and are shaky for a time). Some may even be given anti-thyroid drugs or iodide, too, as temporary relief from the symptoms. After a few months these drugs are stopped, to confirm that the thyroid is now working normally.

Around 50 to 70 per cent of people have normal thyroid function and some goitre shrinkage within six to eight weeks of being given radio-iodine. About 75 per cent are cured after one dose: 20 per cent need a second dose.[7] Only very rarely is a third dose needed. Whether or not a second dose is needed depends largely on the size of the initial dose: a bigger first dose means less likelihood of needing a second. A second dose is not usually considered until at least 6 or even 12 months after the first, as the thyroid can take that time to settle down.

### Problems with Radio-iodine – Real and Imagined

Any treatment that involves radioactivity invokes fear. The first question to be raised is always 'Could it cause cancer?' The facts are very plain. No large-scale study has shown any link between radio-iodine treatment for thyrotoxicosis and subsequent thyroid cancer. The largest of these studies was the Thyrotoxicosis Follow-up Project of the

National Institutes of Health in the United States.[8] It compared 21,714 people treated with radio-iodine with almost 13,000 people given surgery or anti-thyroid drugs. All had thyrotoxicosis. Not only was there no increase in thyroid cancer in the radio-iodine group during the eight years of follow-up, they actually had fewer cancers than the others. Presumably the radiation had destroyed cells with the potential to become cancerous.

One criticism of that study was that it was too short, but two more studies, one in Scandinavia with a follow-up of 13 years, and one from Rochester, Minnesota, with a follow-up of 15 years, found no increase in thyroid cancer in people given radio-iodine.[9] This last study found no increase in any form of cancer after radio-iodine, and other studies have confirmed that there is no risk of leukaemia after radio-iodine for thyrotoxicosis.[10]

These studies were in adults. The long-term effects of radio-iodine in children and young adults are less clear cut. In a 1974 study there were more than the expected number of thyroid adenomas (benign tumours) in adults who had had radio-iodine as children or adolescents.[11] However, in three much larger studies of children who had had radio-iodine, followed up for up to 14 years, there were no increases in cases of thyroid cancer, leukaemia or other cancers.[12] Nor, to settle another worry, was there any problem with future pregnancies, birth and children in the girls.

Despite these reassuring studies, because of an earlier (1959) study report of the development of nodules in the thyroids of three of 18 children given radio-iodine,[13] it is rarely given to children. They are usually treated with anti-thyroid drugs instead. The watershed for deciding on radio-iodine or anti-thyroid drugs appears to be late adolescence. Over that age, most thyroid specialists now prefer to use radio-iodine.

*Pregnancy*
Pregnant women, or women who think they may possibly be pregnant, must never be given radio-iodine. So before any woman of child-bearing age is given radio-iodine there must be a negative pregnancy test or a very recent menstrual period, or she must be prepared to state that she is not sexually active. She may even be asked to sign a declaration to the latter fact.

There is good reason for this. If radio-iodine is given after the 10th week of pregnancy the thyroid in the developing fetus may be irreparably damaged, and the baby born with severe hypothyroidism. There is, happily, some evidence that giving radio-iodine before the 10th week probably does no harm and the baby will eventually be born with a normal thyroid.[14]

Thyrotoxic women who are pregnant are offered anti-thyroid drugs as the treatment of choice. PTU is usually chosen because less of it crosses the placenta into the fetus, but methimazole and carbimazole are also used. The doses of the drugs are kept low, to minimize any effect on the fetus. As thyrotoxicosis usually improves during pregnancy, the dose can usually be cut further and even stopped in many cases. At such low doses the baby is not affected at birth, but the mother must be followed closely in the first few weeks afterwards, because her thyrotoxicosis can become more severe again.

In the past, anti-thyroid drugs were not given to nursing mothers, in case they harmed the baby, but this seems over-cautious. Very little drug gets into the breastmilk, and the consensus is now that mothers can continue to breastfeed, providing that the baby's thyroid function is monitored while they do so.


*Future Damage to Children?*
Another concern often expressed by younger women is whether their dose of radio-iodine may affect their genes, so that their children may be affected. Because the radio-iodine is excreted through the bladder, the ovaries do receive some irradiation, but it is calculated as no more than would be received by other X-ray procedures such as a barium enema or an intravenous pyelogram (done to investigate kidney problems). Any increase in genetic abnormalities that may be caused by radio-iodine has been calculated at under three in one hundred thousand. This is far fewer than the genetic abnormalities that happen spontaneously (eight in one thousand).[15] These calculations are supported by the absence of any abnormalities in the 86 children of 43 women who had had radio-iodine as children themselves,[16] and in another 33 children of women who had received radio-iodine as young adults.[17]

There is no evidence, therefore, that radio-iodine puts either the patient herself or her offspring into any danger, provided that it is not given during the pregnancy. It is probably reasonable, however, for women to avoid getting pregnant for three to six months after being given it.

### Some Sensible Precautions
Despite all this reassurance, it is usual to protect close family members against unnecessary contact with radioactivity. Most of the radioactivity is expelled in the urine, so that the patient should be sure to flush and clean the toilet herself. The saliva is slightly radioactive for several days, so for a few days after the dose the patient should not share food or drink with others, particularly their children, and should avoid kissing them.

### Some After-effects of Radio-iodine
Some people feel nauseated for a while after taking radio-iodine. Others have a transient pain in the front of the neck, probably due to a minor thyroid inflammation. This pain responds well to aspirin.

The most severe side-effect is, paradoxically, a sudden worsening of the thyrotoxicosis. This is because the radiation-damaged thyroid suddenly releases its stores of thyroid hormone into the circulation, raising the blood levels of T3 and T4, which makes the symptoms worse. It can be disconcerting for the patient, and sometimes for the doctor, who may have to deal with the nightmare of a thyrotoxic storm (see page 97).

Because of this possibility, people with severe thyrotoxicosis, those who are elderly or those who have heart problems are usually given a course of anti-thyroid drugs for a few days before radio-iodine treatment. These drugs block any release of thyroid hormone into the circulation and keep the patient in a calm, not 'stormy', state.

Very occasionally, radio-iodine has been reported as making eye symptoms (see page 105) worse. Some experts prefer to give patients with eye problems cortisone-like steroids just after the radio-iodine dose to prevent such a reaction.

### Who Gets Radio-iodine?
To summarize: radio-iodine is used as the main treatment of most adults with thyrotoxicosis, at least in North America. In Europe and Japan, the first-line treatment remains the anti-thyroid drugs in younger adults, radio-iodine being reserved mainly for middle-aged

and older patients. The trend, however, in countries outside North America is towards more use of radio-iodine and less use of anti-thyroid drugs. A very specific use of radio-iodine is for 'solitary thyroid nodules' which over-produceT4 andT3, leading to thyrotoxicosis. The radio-iodine is picked up specifically by the nodules, and hardly at all by the rest of the thyroid, so that the nodule is selectively destroyed. People with such nodules treated in this way very rarely become hypothyroid afterwards, because the normal thyroid gland remains intact.

## Surgery forThyrotoxicosis

Surgery is the oldest way to treat thyrotoxicosis. The surgeon who first developed it in its modern form, Professor Kocher, was awarded the Nobel Prize for it as long ago as 1909. His operation is called *subtotal thyroidectomy*. Most of both lobes are removed, along with the isthmus (see Chapter One), leaving just a rim of each lobe to produce a small fraction of thyroid hormone.Thyroid surgeons are extremely careful to leave a horizontal scar that neatly disappears into a fold of the neck, so that it is almost invisible to anyone without knowledge of thyroid surgery.

In the past, removing the thyroid was fraught with danger. Just manipulating the gland during surgery could release an excess of thyroxine into the circulation, making the patient much worse, and even causing thyroid storm (see page 97). It was only when doctors learned to avoid this by giving anti-thyroid drugs beforehand that this often fatal complication was prevented. Today's thyroid surgery is exceptionally safe: by 1984 the experts were reporting near zero mortality rates post-operatively.[18]

However, the surgery does carry other risks. One is damage to the nerve to the larynx (voicebox), which can leave the person with a permanently hoarse voice, and the other is accidental removal of the parathyroid glands which lie close to the thyroid. These glands control the body's calcium levels. Loss of the parathyroid glands can lead to lifelong problems with calcium balance, which can be difficult to manage even these days. Even in expert hands, around 1 per cent of subtotal thyroidectomies are beset by one or other of these very worrying complications, so it is vital that the surgeon is a real expert, whose main interest is in thyroid surgery. This is particularly important now that anti-thyroid drugs and radio-iodine are the main treatments: there are fewer specialist thyroid surgeons than there were, and they are getting fewer still.

Other, thankfully now very rare, complications include bleeding from, and infection in, the wound, which can make the eventual scar more obvious. People who know that when they cut themselves they form 'keloid' scars (raised, thickened scar tissue) should not have surgery, as the resulting scar can be unsightly.

Today, surgery is the third choice for most patients with thyrotoxicosis. It is restricted largely to children and teenagers who have reacted badly to anti-thyroid drugs and are unsuitable for radio-iodine, to pregnant women, people with large goitres, and people who do not wish to have radio-iodine. In today's open medical climate, the surgeon and thyroid physician will discuss the pros and cons of all the treatments with the patient before the decision is made – and the patient plays her part in that decision.

The correct pre-operative preparation makes a big difference to its outcome. For many years surgeons have given patients around four to six weeks of treatment with an anti-thyroid drug to 'cool the thyroid down' before operating. Today, some surgeons use instead a beta-blocking agent in a high enough dose to lower the resting heart rate to below 80 beats per minute. Which of the two treatment regimens is better is a matter for debate. I am inclined to trust the surgeons in my own area, who still tend to use the anti-thyroid drugs (mostly carbimazole) and only use the beta-blocker method if they need to operate quickly. The difference between them is that the anti-thyroid drug makes the patient euthyroid (with a normal – neither overactive nor underactive – thyroid) on the day of surgery: the beta-blocker does not. Trials have shown that the beta-blocker method leads to more post-operative complications like fever and a fast heartbeat ('tachycardia') than the anti-thyroid drugs.

Removing most of the thyroid gland does not always provide the ideal outcome – a normal thyroid state. In different series of patients, between 10 and 60 per cent become hypothyroid (having an underactive thyroid), with around 3 per cent becoming hypothyroid in each succeeding year. This is why many people need to take thyroid hormone treatment after their operation. Whether or not they become hypothyroid depends on how much thyroid gland has been removed during the operation, and on the reason for their thyrotoxicosis in the first place. The natural history of some forms of Graves' disease is to become, eventually, hypothyroid.

On the other hand, around 5 per cent of people undergoing sub-total thyroidectomy become thyrotoxic (with an overactive thyroid) again, often many years later. In one study, 43 per cent of the reported recurrences happened more than five years after the surgery.[19] It seems that the overactive thyroid can recover its overactive habit even after nine-tenths of it has been removed. People who become thyrotoxic again are offered radio-iodine.

# Chapter Six

# Treating an Underactive Thyroid

The successful treatment of hypothyroidism was one of the biggest medical achievements of the nineteenth century. By 1888 the condition of myxoedema had already been linked with low thyroid gland activity.[1] We are lucky that treatments have moved on since those days, when patients were being given half a sheep's thyroid, lightly fried and minced (with currant jelly!) once a week.[2] Eventually this treatment was replaced by thyroid powder and tablets, and then, after the chemical structure of thyroxine was worked out, by purified thyroxine (T4).

How much and how often thyroxine should be given depends on the person's age and on whether he or she also suffers other illnesses. It is usual to start with 0.05 milligrams per day in young or middle-aged adults with no health problems apart from their thyroid underactivity. The dose is then raised each month by 0.025 milligrams per day until it reaches 0.1 milligram per day. After four to six weeks on this dose, the blood T4 and thyroid-stimulating hormone (TSH) levels are then measured, and the person's thyroid state and symptoms are reassessed.

Whether the dose is kept at 0.1 milligram from then onwards depends on the person's symptoms and the results of the blood tests. The aim is to keep blood T4 levels in or slightly above the normal range, and the TSH level within the normal range. If this is not the case (if for example the T4 level is low and the TSH level is high), there are two possible explanations:

1. The person is not taking her thyroxine (T4).
2. For some reason the person's digestive system is not absorbing the thyroxine.

The first explanation is far more common than the second.

In older people suspected of having heart disease, and in people of any age who are known to have heart disease, thyroxine treatment is started much more carefully, and the dose raised more slowly. This is because giving thyroxine increases the metabolic rate – so that the heart rate and the force of the heartbeat rise, giving the heart more work to do. If the heart is on the edge of failure because of disease, say of the coronary arteries or because of a fault in its rhythm ('arrhythmia'), then adding thyroxine in too high a dose too quickly can push the heart over the edge into failure. People with angina (pain in the heart due to coronary heart disease) may find their angina is worsening, and heart attacks and even sudden death have been put down to initial and subsequent doses of thyroxine being too high.

So in older people with hypothyroidism or those with suspect hearts, the starting dose of thyroxine is usually 0.0125 or 0.025 milligrams, and the increases are again only by 0.0125 or 0.025 milligrams every four to six weeks. Even then, the doctor increases the dose only after carefully evaluating the person's heart and level of hypothyroidism. This may mean keeping her slightly hypothyroid for a while, rather than taking the risk of worsening her heart disease. Follow-up in these early stages is usually every two or three weeks, rather than once a month.

Some people's hypothyroidism is only found after a heart attack or during a severe attack of angina. In people in such circumstances with a normal thyroid it is usual to perform an immediate coronary bypass, or a balloon angioplasty, or to insert a 'stent' in the blocked coronary artery.[3] Operating quickly reduces the risks of sudden death and severe heart damage by around 40 per cent. This benefit applies equally to people with hypothyroidism: several studies show that they are at no more risk than people with normal thyroids when undergoing surgery, provided that the cardiac surgeon or cardiologist knows about the hypothyroid state.[4]

Most people eventually settle on a T4 dose of 0.05 or 0.1 milligrams thyroxine per day, although some need as much as 0.25 milligrams. Each person is different, so that what is correct for one person is not necessarily correct for another. What is aimed for is the dose that keeps the person feeling normal and that keeps the TSH level in the normal range. Under-treated people tend to have TSH levels higher than the upper limit of normal, and still feel a bit slow mentally and physically. Over-treated people may develop an abnormal heart rhythm, heart failure or angina, and the 'shakes', excess appetite and anxiety typical of thyrotoxicosis.

However, not all the symptoms that people may think are caused by their underactive thyroid are necessarily cured by thyroxine treatment. Even weeks after starting thyroxine, many women still feel tired all the time, lack energy and vitality, and are constipated. If their blood TSH and T4 levels are normal, they have to look to other illnesses (often depression) for their symptoms, rather than their thyroid glands. It is often very difficult to persuade them that simply increasing their thyroxine dose will not work.

People whose hypothyroidism is secondary to pituitary problems (see page 69) have extra problems when they start treatment. They must be tested for deficiency in other hormones, such as cortisone, before they start their thyroxine treatment. Giving thyroxine alone may make them more ill, as their cortisone deficiency becomes more apparent. They are usually given cortisone replacement therapy at the same time as the thyroxine is started. Their thyroxine dose is similar to that in people with the usual hypothyroidism, but, of course, their doctors cannot use blood levels of TSH (which they cannot produce) as a measure of how well they are doing.

People who have become hypothyroid after radio-iodine or surgery for thyrotoxicosis (see Chapter Five) may need less thyroxine than people with hypothyroidism due to thyroid disease, mainly because they usually are still producing some thyroxine in the remaining thyroid tissue.

A very small number of people cannot absorb thyroxine from pills very well. Most are already known to have a small bowel disorder that stops them digesting foods ('malabsorption syndrome'). They usually resolve their thyroid problem by taking a slightly larger dose of thyroxine than normal.

If people without obvious malabsorption problems need unusually high thyroxine doses to keep their symptoms of hypothyroidism at bay, it raises the suspicion that they are not taking their treatment regularly enough. This suspicion will be supported by checking their levels of both T4 and TSH. If levels of both are raised, it is because they have taken a thyroxine dose just before the clinic measurement (hence the high T4) – the high TSH level tells us that normally their T4 level is low. So if you are erratic in your medicine-taking, be sure that your sins will be found out!

Occasionally, as in myxoedema coma or very severe hypothyroidism, the illness can be life-threatening and needs rapid correction. In such cases thyroid specialists use tri-iodothyronine (T3, liothyronine, Tertroxin) rather than or along with thyroxine, to get the fastest possible result. T3 is absorbed faster than T4, and is probably the active hormone

(T4, thyroxine, is converted into T3 in the body, and it is T3 that produces the thyroid effects. See page 20). However, the rapid action of T3 is not necessary in the usual person with hypothyroidism, and is marginally more likely (because it is so rapidly active) to affect the heart. It is therefore the second choice thyroid hormone, reserved for the very rare people who do not respond to thyroxine, or for emergencies in specialized hospital units.

A caution about taking other drugs alongside thyroxine. Ciprofloxacin is a popular antibiotic for chest and urinary infections. A cautionary note about it's prescription alongside thyroxine in people with thyroid deficiency. Taken together ciprofloxacin can prevent the uptake of the thyroxine and precipitate a severe low-thyroid state.

Two cases were reported in the British Medical Journal.[5] They were older women admitted to hospital for infections, and had been taking thyroxine for hypothyroidism for years. Until admission to hospital they had normal thyroid function. After three and four weeks respectively of ciprofloxacin treatment their thyroid function 'dived', they were clinically hypothyroid despite maintaining their daily thyroxine doses. Their treatment was changed so that the drugs were given six hours apart, their thyroid function returned to normal. When ciprofloxacin and thyroxine were given simultaneously to these women, the antibiotic prevented the thyroxine from being absorbed. Other drugs may interfere with the body's uptake of thyroxine. These include antacids, laxatives, colestipol and cholestyramine (for lowering cholesterol levels), iron tablets (mainly ferrous sulphate), sucralfate (for stomach and duodenal ulcers) and raloxifene (for osteoporosis).

What should you do if you have to take thyroxine alongside other drugs? For many drugs there should be no problem taking the two together. To ensure there is no interaction set out a specific time to take your thyroxine that is several hours different from the time you take the other drugs. Most medicines are prescribed as once-daily treatments making it easy to organize. If your thyroxine tablets aren't working as well as they used to, and you have recently started a new treatment for another complaint, do ask your doctor about interactions. It is simple to check and needs only a single blood test for TSH and T3 levels. Usually it is enough to space out the doses to make sure that you get the benefit from the thyroxine you have swallowed.

# Part Four
# Problems Associated with Thyroid Disease

# Chapter Seven

# Thyroid Emergencies: 'Storm' and Coma

In most people with thyroid problems, their illness develops gradually, so that there is no emergency. Their doctors can take time to investigate them, and start treatment almost at their leisure, knowing that there is no immediate danger to life.

However, both the overactive and underactive forms of thyroid disease can turn dramatically for the worse, so that people with them need emergency treatment to save their lives. When an overactive thyroid turns dramatically worse, the problem is called thyrotoxic storm. When an underactive thyroid worsens, it can cause myxoedema coma. Both problems are rare – most general practitioners will see one or two cases in a lifetime of practice – but this book would be incomplete without describing them.

## Thyrotoxic Storm

In thyrotoxic storm, the symptoms of the illness suddenly become much worse. Most people who develop it are already under treatment for thyrotoxicosis (although it may have been inadequate). It starts with a very high fever and a very fast heart rate – so fast that the patient feels a lot of discomfort in the chest. It soon progresses to emotional swings, with anxiety and fear, restlessness, agitation, confusion, then what appears to be an acute mental illness, with hallucinations. Finally the patient lapses into coma, and can die from heart failure and shock.

What causes people to develop this massively overactive thyroid gland is still unknown. It is not just a matter of a sudden release of an excess of thyroid hormones: there may also be a change in the body's cells that makes them temporarily much more sensitive to the thyroid hormone that is produced. We do know that it may be brought on by an infection, or by a serious accident, or severe emotional stress. It has been reported in women just after childbirth, in people who have suddenly stopped their anti-thyroid drug treatment, as a complication of poorly controlled diabetes, and after a stroke or thrombosis in the lung.

## Treatment

The treatment is immediate admission to hospital for intensive care. Patients with thyrotoxic storm are given anti-thyroid drugs to lower thyroid hormone production, but they must also be given treatments to lower the fever, to combat the heart failure and slow down the heart, and to restore the low blood pressure (the cause of shock) to normal. The cause of the 'storm' (such as diabetes or infection) will be sought, and corrected if possible. This book is not the place to go into such treatments in detail, but in experienced hands there is usually a dramatic improvement within 12 hours that leads to complete recovery within three to four days. Even in hospital, published death rates have varied from 10 to 75 per cent.[1] Outside hospital they approach 100 per cent.

## Myxoedema Coma

Myxoedema coma is a rare condition that is seen more often in the winter than in the summer, raising the suspicion that it is possibly an extreme reaction to cold. It is also linked to lung infections such as pneumonia and acute bronchitis, strokes and heart failure. It may also be an unusual side-effect of drugs, mainly sedatives, antidepressants and tranquillizers, or even anaesthetics given during surgery.

People who develop myxoedema coma may have been hypothyroid for some time, but the diagnosis has been missed, or they have not consulted their doctors. On the other hand, some have known they were hypothyroid but stopped their thyroid hormone treatment. Others may have had surgery or radio-iodine treatment for previous thyrotoxicosis, then dropped out of their doctors' follow-up and become hypothyroid, unknown to themselves.

Whatever the underlying cause, people with myxoedema coma first become very lethargic, and slowly drift into a stupor (a sleepy, confused state) before becoming deeply unconscious. They may be found unconscious by a neighbour or other visitor in their home. Many get into this state because they live alone and have no one to notice their deterioration.

People in myxoedema coma have dry, coarse and scaly skin, a

puffy face, sparse and coarse hair, a yellowish tinge to the skin, and a tongue that may be so large that it protrudes from the mouth. They may be obviously choking on it. They breathe very slowly, only a few times a minute. The pulse is often difficult to feel, and is very slow, often around 40 to 50 beats per minute. But the feature that is most obvious to the people finding them is how cold they feel. The normal body temperature is around 37 degrees centigrade. In myxoedema coma it can drop to 27 degrees centigrade, well below the lowest reading on a normal clinical thermometer. A special low-reading thermometer is needed to get the true picture of how cold the person really is. In the depth of a cold winter, in a cold room, it is easy to assume that this is a simple case of hypothermia and the true diagnosis can be missed, with fatal consequences if thyroid replacement treatment is not started. On the other hand, myxoedema coma can strike at any time, and it is unlikely to be confused with hypothermia at warmer times of year.

It is vital to make the correct diagnosis, because the treatment for myxoedema coma is to give thyroxine – and this could kill an elderly person with a normal thyroid and true hypothermia. Pointers to myxoedema coma, rather than other causes of coma such as stroke or hypothermia, include the very slow heartbeat; the cold, dry skin (without any previous or present shivering); the swollen tongue; the very light and slow breathing; and perhaps a scar on the throat indicating a previous thyroid operation. Knowledge that the person has been taking thyroid drugs or a sedative (which are sometimes linked with myxoedema coma) is another strong extra indication.

## Treatment

Myxoedema coma must be treated urgently: untreated, death follows very quickly. So it needs emergency admission to intensive care. The treatment includes breathing support, usually with a mechanical respirator, control of blood oxygen and carbon dioxide levels, normalizing the blood levels of salts and glucose, bringing the blood pressure up to normal, and warming the patient up with blankets. Steroids are usually given, along with thyroid hormone replacement. The type and amount of thyroid hormone given is still debated by the experts: it is enough here to state that eitherT3 orT4 is given by injection under close supervision.

Even with such vigorous treatment, some people, especially the elderly, do not survive myxoedema coma. The first 48 hours of treatment are crucial. Most people are back to normal consciousness within that time: those still in coma after two days are unlikely to survive.

Sadly, some people are precipitated into myxoedema coma by a well-meaning health care team. Older people already known to be hypothyroid, who may have been neglecting their thyroid hormone treatment, are sometimes brought into hospital for other reasons. The stress of having tests, or being put on a drip, or being given sleeping tablets to help them through the noisy hospital night may all push them over the edge from a poor thyroid state into coma. So anyone with hypothyroidism who is asked to go into hospital for any reason should make their thyroid condition clear to the staff, and make sure that they take their regular thyroxine dose every day.

Signs of impending myxoedema coma in someone at home include psychological changes. They may become disorientated (not knowing where they are or what time it is), depressed or paranoid (accusing their carers of hating them or stealing from them), or they may hallucinate (this last is termed myxoedema madness). They lose their recent memory and may even have amnesia, forgetting who they are, and become unusually clumsy and shaky, before becoming sleepy, then comatose. About a quarter of them have fits. All of these symptoms disappear dramatically if they are given their thyroid hormone dose.

# Chapter Eight

# Behavioural and Psychological Problems

Ever since they were first recognized in the eighteenth and nineteenth centuries, thyroid problems have been linked with psychological disorders. In Caleb Parry's paper on what we now call thyrotoxicosis in 1825, he blamed the illness on a young woman's fear when trapped in a runaway wheelchair.[1] The idea that hyperthyroidism was due to stress was still being mooted more than a hundred years later. Here is Dr E. Moschowitz, writing in 1930:

> Those influences that tend towards conflict and sensitization of the individual will breed Graves' syndrome, which in the final analysis is a social disease and a product of higher civilization.

It is true that many people with thyrotoxicosis are anxious, often weepy and unhappy, have massive mood swings, cannot sleep and feel they are not as intellectually able as they were. Early in the illness they lose their ability to concentrate: they become restless and are quick to anger. They speak and think too fast. In fact the illness is sometimes confused with mania, the 'high' phase of manic depression. The extreme form of this is the thyrotoxic storm mentioned in the previous chapter, in which patients can become delirious and very agitated, and needing of psychiatric, as well as physical care.

Happily, thyrotoxic storm is now very rare, but minor degrees of psychiatric disturbance are much more common, and need understanding and good management. However, it is clear that the old idea that thyrotoxicosis is the *result* of some form of psychiatric illness or psychological or social problem is wrong. Many modern studies have shown that there is no particular personality or mental trait that predisposes people to developing thyroid disease. Even claims that psychological stress may precipitate thyrotoxicosis are anecdotal and have not been substantiated in modern studies. It seems that the thyrotoxicosis, the excessive amount of circulating thyroid hormones, causes the psychological and psychiatric symptoms in people, and not the other way round.

The proof of this is that the successful return of the thyrotoxic state to normal (the 'euthyroid' state) quickly resolves the mental symptoms. Anxiety, agitation, emotional problems and muscle tension all return to normal levels once the patient becomes euthyroid. People feel, too, as they return to normal, that they are getting back their lost reasoning powers.

There is usually no need for drugs or other psychological or psychiatric treatment, except sometimes in the acute stage, in some patients who are excessively agitated. Then perhaps a beta-blocking agent may help to reduce palpitations and anxiety.

In fact, if someone with thyrotoxicosis is misdiagnosed as having a psychiatric illness, such as mania (sometimes the two seem similar), giving an anti-mania drug can be positively dangerous. For example, such drugs can mask the thyrotoxic state, so that the eye symptoms can worsen and damage vision. One anti-manic drug, haloperidol, has even been reported as precipitating thyrotoxic storm in a patient misdiagnosed as manic when the true problem was thyrotoxicosis.[2]

The main need for anyone with thyrotoxicosis and mental and psychological problems is not for drugs, but skilled help from someone who understands them and can give them insight into their mental state, so that they know that it is just a passing phase caused by the thyroid abnormality. Enthusiasm and encouragement can achieve much more than drugs.

The psychological symptoms in adult hypothyroidism start as poorly-defined complaints, such as weakness, loss of reasoning power, slowing of thought processes, poor concentration and poor recent memory. As the illness proceeds, the memory loss goes further back, it becomes more difficult to do everyday things, and the patient begins to lack concern for others, is less interested in what is going on around her, and becomes less able to learn new tasks and skills.

In the later stages, vision is less accurate, so that the person with myxoedema may start 'seeing things' and behave bizarrely. Eventually there is a permanent drowsiness, so that people find it difficult to arouse her. She starts sleeping for most of the day, and may eventually lapse into coma – the myxoedema coma described in the last chapter.

The picture is therefore of slowing of thought and speech, poor attention, inability to concentrate, and a loss of interest in everything worthwhile and everyone close to the sufferer. It is not surprising that two common misdiagnoses in hypothyroidism, particularly when the obvious changes in appearance may not be present, are dementia and depression.

This is why it is vital for everyone labelled as depressed or demented to have blood tests to ensure that their thyroid state is normal. A person with the mental symptoms described in the paragraphs above, who also has a high TSH and low T3 and T4 levels, must be treated as myxoedematous. Treatment with the appropriate thyroid hormone will dramatically improve things – and dispel the fear of dementia and depression.

This link between hypothyroidism and depression, and its cure using thyroid hormone, was recognized as long ago as 1892 by Dr C Shaw, in his 'case of myxoedema with restless melancholia treated by injections of thyroid juice' in the British Medical Journal.[3] Sadly, some cases are still misdiagnosed to this day.

The treatment is adequate doses of thyroid hormone (usually T4). It is only very rarely that drugs to treat the mental illness are needed. However, on the rare occasions when a patient has both myxoedema and a history of manic depression, then great care must be taken in choosing the dose of the anti-depressant drug.

Some people with severe hypothyroidism may have heart problems that are worsened by giving certain types of anti-depressant or anti-manic drugs. They must have their heart function monitored in the early stages of thyroid hormone treatment.

# Chapter Nine

# When Thyroid Disease Affects the Eyes

Ask people in the street what they know about thyroid problems and it is odds on that they will say it causes protruding eyes. Technically, the bulging eye problem is called 'ophthalmopathy'. It is often the most distressing part of overactive thyroid disease (thyrotoxicosis). People with the beginnings of ophthalmopathy complain of a gritty feeling in the eyes and a pressure behind them, as if something is pushing them forwards and out of their sockets. Their eyes often fill with tears, their vision becomes blurred and they often see double.

The type of blurring is very important. If it is cleared by blinking, then it is just due to the film of tears on the eyeball. If it is cleared by closing one eye, then the problem is a slight muscle imbalance between the two eyes that is not yet enough to cause frank double vision. But if the blurred vision continues for weeks and persists even when one eye is closed, particularly if colours are not as bright as they used to be, this may be caused by pressure on the optic nerve – the nerve that carries the signals of sight to the brain. Tests will probably show, too, that the peripheral vision (what we can see to the side of us) is also affected. This last type of blurring is the beginning of 'optic neuropathy' and should alert patient and doctor to the need for urgent treatment to save the eyesight.

The most common complaint of people with early Graves' disease is that they look as if they are staring. The 'stare' comes from a combination of two problems: their eyelids are too wide open, and the eyeballs are being pushed forwards in their sockets by swelling of the muscles and fatty tissues behind them. Whatever the cause, it is often difficult to close the eyes completely; this leaves the front of the eyes (the cornea) dry and inflamed. It is vital for people with such eye problems to avoid smoke and draughts, which can further irritate the cornea.

The double vision arises because the muscles that move the eye around in the socket are less able to co-ordinate with each other than they should be. It may or may not be obvious as a squint.

105

Graves' ophthalmopathy usually worsens slowly, over the first six months or so of the disease. It then stays at roughly the same severity for many months, before finally, in most people, recovering, again slowly. It is during the initial worsening phase, when corneal ulcers' pressure on the optic nerve threatens blindness, that urgent treatment may be needed. After that, even though the condition is getting no worse, the muscles controlling the eye movements may become scarred, leaving the patient with a squint and severe double vision. So it is important for the doctor to assess the eye status correctly and take the appropriate action to prevent permanent damage to the eyesight and the person's appearance.

The questions such people will be asked include:

● How long have you had the eye symptoms?
● Do you have eye pain, excessive tears, blurred vision or double vision?
● Do you shy away from bright light?
● Are the symptoms worsening or stable?
● Can you tolerate them, or do you desperately need relief from them?

The doctor will then examine the condition of the cornea, the optic nerve (seen through an ophthalmoscope) and the muscles of eye movement, and test the eyes for colour vision and visual fields (the breadth of sideways and vertical vision).

## Treatment

All treatment of ophthalmopathy aims to protect the eyes from further deterioration until either the condition resolves itself or it can be corrected by surgical or other means.

The first and simplest step is to wear tinted glasses out of doors to protect the eye surface from dust and wind. Instilling artificial tears into the eyes at frequent intervals helps to relieve the constant feeling of grit in the eye. Some people find a protective eye patch or taping the eyelids together at night helps to protect the cornea.

Medical treatment for ophthalmopathy includes high doses of cortisone-like steroids: they often relieve eye pain, dislike of bright light (photophobia), swelling of the tissues around the eye and redness, but they are less effective against the eye protrusion ('proptosis') or the problem with the eye muscles. Some experts recommend steroid injections around the back of the eyes, but many people refuse them. In severe cases, combining steroids with radiotherapy to the back of the eyes and the immune suppressant drug cyclosporin (more often used after organ transplants to prevent rejection) has been successful.

There is argument about whether radio-iodine may make the eye symptoms worse in some patients with thyrotoxicosis. As radio-iodine is often used during the period when the condition is worsening anyway, there is no real evidence to support this notion.

Radiotherapy to the back of the eyes (to reduce the swollen tissues behind the eyeballs) has had mixed reports, ranging from poor responses to very good responses, but the consensus is that it rarely improves the proptosis or the double vision.

Surgery can help a lot. The most common operation is 'orbital decompression' in which parts of the wall of the orbit (the bony sockets in which the eyes lie) are removed to give the thickened soft tissues behind the eye more room. There are many different techniques, but they all aim to reduce the pressure behind the eye and can greatly relieve all the symptoms and the person's appearance. Double vision that persists after decompression or after the ophthalmopathy has resolved can be cured by shortening or weakening the appropriate eye muscles. It is usual for the surgeon to wait for at least two months after decompression, to allow the eye muscles to settle, before a muscle operation is considered. Where the person has not had a decompression, the surgeon extends that wait for at least six months after steroids have been stopped, to make sure that there will be no further natural recovery that would eliminate the need for surgery.

Finally, once the decompression and the eye muscle surgery are over, the surgeon may wish to re-position the eyelids to improve the person's appearance. This involves bringing the eyelids closer together, so that the whites of the eyes are not seen all round the pupil. It can be extremely successful, giving great satisfaction to the patient – and the surgeon.

# Chapter Ten

# Thyrotoxicosis Factitia: When the Patient Is the Cause

Sadly, a book on thyroid disease would not be complete without mention of 'factitious thyrotoxicosis', or thyrotoxicosis factitia. In patients with this illness, the thyroid and pituitary glands are normal, but they have brought on their overactive thyroid state themselves, by swallowing thyroxine tablets.

Why they should do so has puzzled doctors ever since thyroid hormone treatment was started for hypothyroid states over a hundred years ago.[1] During the early and middle years of the twentieth century, first thyroid gland extracts, then purified thyroxine, were given not just for thyroid gland disease, but also for completely unrelated problems such as obesity, irregular periods, infertility and baldness.

Naturally such treatments were useless, but it used to be common for doctors, and often the patients themselves, to raise the dose of thyroid hormone in the mistaken belief that higher doses might actually work. The result was thyrotoxicosis – hyperthyroidism due to far too high a level of thyroxine in the blood. And this form of overactive thyroid often went unrecognized in the enthusiasm the patient (and sometimes the doctor) felt for the treatment.

Today, good general practitioners are very careful never to prescribe thyroxine for any condition except where there is a proven need for it. This is particularly true of people who wish to use thyroxine to lose weight. To do that, they must put themselves into a hyperthyroid state, and this is hardly a healthy way to go about slimming.

However, knowing that taking excessive doses of thyroxine can cause harm does not stop some people from doing so. Many feel the risks are outweighed by the weight loss – but that is temporary, and it is soon gained again, even when they continue to take the thyroxine. All that happens is that they eat more, and their metabolism is shifted on to a higher gear – that accelerator pedal mentioned in the Introduction is stuck down on the boards.

Others have more subtle motives for taking an excess of thyroxine when they do not need it. Many have some medical or nursing training, and find that making themselves thyrotoxic by swallowing thyroxine makes them the focus of medical attention, in a form of Munchausen's syndrome. Baron Munchausen was famous for his outrageous fantasy life and lies: Munchausen's syndrome is a disease brought on deliberately by a patient who desperately craves medical attention. In a tragic twist to this syndrome, mothers sometimes feed thyroxine to their children, making them the victims of 'Munchausen's disease by proxy'. Children have also been known to swallow their parents' thyroxine tablets, making them temporarily thyrotoxic. So thyrotoxicosis should be considered as one possible cause of a sudden illness with fast heartbeat in an overactive, flushed child in a house where there is easy access to thyroxine tablets.

Some people have a more straightforward reason for taking unnecessary thyroxine. They have a financial interest in being ill, receiving insurance money while being off work with the diagnosis of thyrotoxicosis.

Occasionally, thyrotoxicosis factitia happens in people who are taking thyroxine correctly, because they are hypothyroid or have an under-functioning thyroid gland with a goitre, but the dose is too high for them and they swing from a hypothyroid state to a hyperthyroid one. These people, of course, are usually diagnosed quite quickly, as they do not keep their medication a secret.

Making the diagnosis of thyrotoxicosis factitia is relatively simple. A doctor suspecting thyrotoxicosis because the patient is secretly consuming thyroxine will measure the blood level of thyroglobulin (Tg) – the protein to which naturally produced thyroxine is attached in the circulation. In the usual cases of thyrotoxicosis, such as Graves' disease (see page 31), Tg levels are at least normal and usually high. There is no Tg, however, in tablets of thyroxine, so that in thyrotoxicosis caused by swallowing too much thyroxine the blood Tg levels are extremely low or even absent, while the thyroxine levels are exceptionally high.

The problem is then how to face the patient with the diagnosis. As the hormone is usually being taken without the knowledge of family, carers and friends, the doctor can be faced with outright and even righteous denial. And the family can be taken in, often taking sides against the doctor. This can lead to permanent breakdown in the doctor-patient relationship, which is always sad.

So if you are reading this book to understand a relative's condition, do keep in mind the possibility that he or she may be taking thyroxine secretly. It is much more common than you may imagine. The treatment of thyrotoxicosis factitia could not be simpler, however. All that is needed is for the person to stop taking the tablets. This is often harder than it sounds, but if the person does so, he or she will then return to a normal thyroid state, and the blood Tg levels, along with T3 and T4 levels, will return to normal. If these levels do not return to normal, then either the person is still taking thyroxine surreptitiously, or has true thyrotoxicosis. This needs further investigations, which are described in Chapter Three.

# Chapter Eleven

# Thyroid Cancer

At the back of the minds of many people with thyroid disease, both hyper- and hypothyroidism, is the question 'Does it become cancer?' The answer is an unequivocal 'no'. So if you fear that your thyroid disease will turn to cancer, you can rest assured that you have no greater chance of developing thyroid cancer than someone who has never had thyroid disease.

Thyroid cancer is rare. It only accounts for around 1 per cent of all cancers and, because it is usually curable, less than a third of 1 per cent of all cancer deaths. And even this small number of thyroid cancers has arisen mostly in people who have had radiotherapy for other cancers in the neck region, usually many years before. Thyroid cancers have also been reported after exposure to radiation in the environment, the most disastrous cases being in people living in the Marshall Islands in the South Seas, who were affected by the fallout after the 1954 nuclear bomb tests, and in children living near Chernobyl. As mentioned on page 81, there is absolutely no evidence that radio-iodine treatment causes thyroid cancer.

Nor is there any conclusive evidence that any other thyroid disease (such as Graves' disease, myxoedema, thyroiditis or euthyroid goitre) predisposes a person to cancer of the thyroid, despite many studies exploring the possibility. If there is any link, it must be very small, with very few cases.

Cancers of the thyroid start as 'nodules', small discrete lumps within the thyroid that are usually painless, firm and obvious. People come to their doctor because they have found the lump. However, only a tiny proportion of people with thyroid nodules have cancers. About 4 per cent of the population have thyroid nodules at some time in their lives. Only one in a thousand of these nodules is a thyroid cancer.[1] However, this should not lead people to neglect any lump in the neck: among people with a solitary lump (most people with nodules have more than one) around 5 to 10 per cent have a thyroid cancer.

Features that do point to possible cancer include a single, hard lump that seems stuck to the skin above it and/or the tissues beneath it, that is fast growing, and that is associated with a persistently hoarse voice. It usually starts before the age of 14 or after 65 years of age, with enlarged, firm, not tender glands on the same side of the neck, especially in someone who has had radiotherapy to the neck, for another cancer, in the past.

Cancer is diagnosed by a 'fine-needle biopsy', in which a tiny piece of the nodule is removed for microscopic inspection. The procedure takes only a few seconds and there is very little discomfort. The result is reported virtually immediately, and the appropriate treatment started.

Most thyroid cancers are cured by surgery. Some surgeons remove the part of the gland harbouring the tumour, others remove the whole thyroid – there is still debate about which is best. On the whole, it seems safest to remove the whole gland and give the patient thyroxine replacement treatment to deal with the inevitable hypothyroidism that follows. People who have only part of the gland removed for a tumour have a one in five chance of needing the rest removed later for a second cancer.[2]

All thyroid cancers are now treated in centres where the surgeons are operating on the neck, and thyroids, almost exclusively. The surgeon's choice lies among:

1. lumpectomy (removing the nodule and a little tissue around it)
2. partial thyroidectomy (removing the nodule plus more surrounding tissue)
3. subtotal thyroidectomy (removing almost all the thyroid on both sides)
4. hemithyroidectomy (removing the half of the thyroid that has the tumour)
5. total thyroidectomy (removing the whole thyroid)

If you are facing surgery for thyroid cancer, do discuss the options with your surgeon, who will explain the usual practice in his or her unit. The decision on which operation is chosen may depend on age, the microscopic appearance of the tumour (how malignant it looks), whether it is limited to the thyroid gland alone, and its size (whether it is under or over 1.5 centimetres in diameter).

After the surgery you will be left with a light pressure dressing on the neck, and you will be lying with your head and neck raised to minimize the pressure in the neck veins. Most people can swallow liquids by the evening of the day of the operation, can eat normally by the next day, and go home that day or the next.

Most people with thyroid cancers do very well, with a very low rate of recurrences, so if you have had such a cancer, be optimistic. You will always have to return for follow-up checks, but there is no reason to be frightened of the future.

# Questions and Answers

While writing this book, my editors asked about several conditions popularly thought to be linked to thyroid disease. The following paragraphs seek to answer these commonly held beliefs – often, as you shall see, misconceptions.

**Q. Is there any link between thyroid disease and rheumatoid arthritis?**

A. As far as I know, there is no proven connection between thyroid disease and rheumatoid arthritis. Most people with hypothyroidism (underactive thyroid), for example, make very few complaints of arthritis – instead they complain of tiredness, constipation, intolerance to cold, and stiff and aching muscles which they often attribute to 'rheumatism'. However, this is not a true arthritis, but the consequence of the loss of thyroid hormone. The symptoms soon disappear after treatment starts.

Weakness and tingling ('pins and needles') in the hands in those suffering myxoedema (a severe form of underactive thyroid disease) may be due to carpal tunnel syndrome, in which a band of thickened tissue in the wrist compresses the nerves running under it into the hand. This, too, may resolve after starting treatment: a few may need surgery to decompress the nerve.

People with thyrotoxicosis (overactive thyroid disease) are more likely to complain about muscle weakness and wasting of the muscles of the shoulders and the hips: the muscles in these areas may 'fasciculate', or ripple uncontrollably. Very rarely, weakness of the muscles of the trunk and limbs can lead to actual temporary paralysis. These symptoms all disappear after the patient's thyroid function is brought back to normal.

**Q. Can thyroid disease contribute to deafness?**

A. There is no definite evidence, though it is often claimed, of a link between thyroid disease (either hyperthyroidism or hypothyroidism) and tinnitus or deafness.

The three common causes of tinnitus are Meniere's disease (in which the pressure in the inner ear is raised), circulation problems in older age and, more rarely, tumours of the auditory nerve between the ear and the brain. Thyroid disease does not feature in this list. People with myxoedema (underactive thyroid) react slowly to sound, as they do to any other stimulus. That may cause others to think they are deaf, so that they are taken to an ENT department for tests, which are usually negative. They are not in the strict sense deaf.

**Q. Can taking vitamin A help thyroid disease?**

A. There is no evidence that extra vitamin A (carotene) helps either type of thyroid disease, or that either is linked to vitamin A deficiency. However, three different types of anaemia *are* linked to myxoedema.

The first is an iron deficiency anaemia due to loss of blood from excessive menstrual periods ('menorrhagia'), which is usually controlled by thyroid hormone and a few months of iron tablets.

The second is an anaemia simply due to under-production of red blood cells by the bone marrow – it is slowed down by lack of thyroid hormone, just like all other processes in the body. It is corrected simply by giving thyroxine.

The third is a form of pernicious anaemia, linked to antibody disturbances associated with a more general immune problem which also shuts down thyroxine production. It is treated with both thyroxine and injections of vitamin B12.

**Q. Does thyroid disease cause sleep disorders?**

A. People with an overactive thyroid tend to sleep less, but they rarely complain about it. Those with myxoedema often sleep more than normal, during the day as well as at night, but it is others who are bothered by this, not usually themselves. In either case, correcting the thyroid problem corrects the sleep disturbance.

**Q. Is snoring a sign of thyroid disease?**

A. Very rarely. Most snoring is linked to obesity, particularly around the neck, or to blockages in the nasal passages and enlarged tonsils and adenoids. People with myxoedema tend to put on weight, which may be the reason for the apparent link with snoring. However, thyroid disease does not seem to cause snoring *per se*. It can cause a croaky, slurred voice because the vocal cords are thickened and covered with a thick mucus. This, too, improves dramatically with thyroxine treatment.

**Q. Can thyroid disease lead to period problems?**

A. Period problems include menorrhagia (see paragraph above) in myxoedema and very light periods ('oligomenorrhoea') in thyrotoxicosis. Both are corrected with the appropriate thyroid treatment, as is the infertility sometimes associated with thyrotoxicosis.

**Q. How does an underactive thyroid affect the nails and hair?**

A. The nails may thicken and be more rough than normal in myxoedema, and the hair becomes very sparse. Both symptoms gradually improve on the corrective treatment, the nails more slowly than the hair.

**Q. Can drug abuse lead to thyroid problems?**

A. Drug abuse has been claimed to cause either form of thyroid disease, but there is little evidence that it does so.

**Q. Is thyroid disease connected at all with dementia?**

A. Myxoedema has been linked with Alzheimer's disease, mainly because the two are superficially similar in their symptoms. However, the symptoms of myxoedema are reversed by thyroxine; those of Alzheimer's are not. There is no real evidence that having myxoedema predisposes people to Alzheimer's. Myxoedema may be more common in people with Down's syndrome, in which case it should be treated just as vigorously as in the rest of the population.

# Glossary

Anti-thyroid drugs

Drugs used to prevent the formation of T4 and T3 in cases of an overactive thyroid. The main ones are propylthiouracil (PTU) and carbimazole or methimazole

Euthyroid

The normal thyroid state

Hyperthyroid

A condition in which the thyroid gland is overactive

Hypothyroid

A condition in which the thyroid is underactive

Myxoedema

Hypothyroidism with specific facial and skin changes

Myxoedema coma

A very severe, life-threatening form of myxoedema

Parathyroids

Four small pea-like glands whose hormone controls calcium levels in the blood and bone. They lie just behind the thyroid gland, so may be affected by thyroid surgery or irradiation

Radio-iodine ($I^{131}$)

Radioactive iodine, used to reduce the thyroid gland's ability to produce T4 and T3 in people with hyperthyroidism

Thyroidectomy

Surgical removal of the thyroid

Thyroid storm

A very severe form of thyrotoxicosis

Thyrotoxicosis

Hyperthyroidism with specific eye and heart signs

| Thyrotrophin (TSH) | Otherwise known as thyroid-stimulating hormone, it is produced by the pituitary gland in response to low T4 and T3 levels in the blood |
| --- | --- |
| Thyroxine (T4) | The main hormone produced by the thyroid gland |
| Tri-iodothyronine (T3) | The thyroid hormone that produces the main thyroid effects: it is formed from T4 in the tissues to become the active hormone. In medicine form also known as liothyronine and Tertroxin |

# References

## Chapter 2

1. Wespi, H M *et al.*, *Schweiz Medizinische Wochenschrift* vol. 75, 1945, p. 625
2. Konig, M P, *Die Kongenitale Hypothyreose und der Endemische Kretinismus* (Berlin: Springer-Verlag, 1968)
3. Delange, F, in J T Dunn *et al.*, *Towards the eradication of endemic goiter, cretinism and iodine deficiency* (Washington, DC: PAHO Scientific Publication no. 502, 1986, p. 373)
4. Goyens, P *et al.*, 'Selenium deficiency as possible factor in the pathogenesis of myxedematous endemic cretinism', *Acta Endocrinol* vol. 114, 1987, p. 497
5. Oliver, J W, 'Interrelationships between athyreotic and manganese deficient states in rats', *American Journal of Veterinary Research* vol. 37, 1976, p. 597
6. Pharoah, P O D and Hornabrook, R W, 'Endemic cretinism of recent onset in New Guinea', *Lancet* ii, 1973, p. 1038
7. Ermans, A M *et al.*, *Role of cassava in the etiology of endemic goitre and cretinism* (Ottawa: International Development Research Centre, 1980)
8. Clements, F W and Wishart, J W, 'A thyroid-blocking agent in the etiology of endemic goitre', *Metabolism* vol. 5, 1956, p. 623; Gmelin, R and Virtanen, A, 'The enzymic formation of thiocyanate (SCN) from a precursor in Brassica species', *Acta Chemica Scandinavia* vol. 14, 1960, p. 507
9. Suzuki, H *et al.*, 'Endemic coast goitre in Hokkaido, Japan', *Acta Endocrinologica* vol. 50, 1965, p. 161

## Chapter 3

1. Graves, R J, 'Clinical Lectures', *London Medical and Surgical Journal* vol. 7, 1835, p. 516
2. von Basedow, C A, 'Exophthalmos durch Hypertrophie des Zellgewebes in der Augenhohle', *Wochenschr Heilk* vol. 6, 1840, p. 197

3.  Parry, C H, *Collections from the unpublished papers of the late Caleb Hilliel Parry* (vol. 2; London: Underwoods, 1825, p. 111)
4.  Gray J, and Hoffenberg, R, 'Thyrotoxicosis and Stress', *Quarterly Journal of Medicine* vol. 54, 1985, p. 153
5.  Adams, D D and Purves, H D, 'Abnormal responses in the assay of thyrotropin', *Otago Medical School Proceedings* vol. 34, 1956, p. 11
6.  Gray J, and Hoffenberg, R, 'Thyrotoxicosis and Stress', *Quarterly Journal of Medicine* vol. 54, 1985, p. 153
7.  Volpe, R, in L E Braverman, and R D Utiger (eds), *The Thyroid* (J B Lippincott, 1991, p. 654)
8.  Hamilton, C R *et al.*, 'Hyperthyroidism due to thyrotropin producing pituitary chromophobe adenoma', *New England Journal of Medicine* vol. 283, 1970, p. 1077
9.  Hill, S A *et al.*, 'Thyrotrophin-producing pituitary adenomas', *Journal of Neurosurgery* vol. 57, 1982, p. 515
10. Plummer, H S, *American Journal of Medical Science* vol. 146, 1913, p. 790
11. de Quervain, F, in *Mitt Grenz Med Chir* vol. 2, 1904, p. 1
12. Mygind, H, *Journal of Laryngology*, vol. 9 1895, p. 181

# Chapter 4

1.  Gill, Dr W W, 'On a cretinoid state supervening in adult life in women *Transactions of the Clinical Society* vol. 7, 1874, p. 180
2.  Hashimoto, H, *Archive Klinikal Chirurgerie* [in German] vol. 97, 1912, p. 21
3.  Hawkins, B R *et al.*, *Lancet* vol. 8203, 1980, p. 1057
4.  Vople, R (Boca Raton; FL: CRC Press, 1990, p. 73)
5.  Chertow, B S *et al.*, *Acta Endocrinologica* vol. 72, 1973, p. 18; Jayson, M I V *et al.*, *Lancet* vol. 2, 1967, p. 15
6.  Hamburger, J I, in *Controversies in clinical thyroidology* (New York: Springer-Verlag, 1981, p. 21)
7.  Othman, S *et al.*, *Clinical Endocrinology* vol. 32, 1990, p. 559
8.  Cunnien, A J *et al.*, *Journal of Nuclear Medicine* vol. 23, 1982, p. 978
9.  Sridama, V *et al.*, *New England Journal of Medicine* vol. 311, 1984, p. 426

10. Lindstedt, G *et al.*, *British Journal of Psychiatry* vol. 130, 1977, p. 452
11. Mazonson, P D, *American Journal of Medicine* vol. 77, 1984, p. 751
12. Sheehan, H L and Stanfield, J P, *Acta Endocrinologica Copenhagen* vol. 37, 1961, p. 479

## Chapter 5

1. Astwood, E B, *Journal of the American Medical Association* vol. 122, 1943, p. 78
2. Cooper, D S, *New England Journal of Medicine* vol. 311, 1984, p. 1353
3. Lippe, B M, *Journal of Endocrinological Metabolism* vol. 64, 1987, p. 1241
4. Sugrue, D *et al.*, *Quarterly Journal of Medicine* vol. 439, 1980, p. 51
5. Amino, N *et al.*, *Journal of Endocrinology and Metabolism* vol. 55, 1982, p. 108
6. Wenzel, K W, *Journal of Clinical Endocrinology and Metabolism* vol. 6, 1983, p. 389
7. Holm, L E, *Acta Radiologica* vol. 20, 1981, p. 162
8. Dobyns, B M *et al.*, *Journal of Clinical Endocrinology and Metabolism* vol. 38, 1974, p. 96
9. Holm, L E *et al.*, *New England Journal of Medicine* vol. 303, 1980, p. 188; Hoffman, D A *et al.*, *American Journal of Epidemiology* vol. 115, 1982, p. 243
10. Saenger, E L *et al.*, *Journal of the American Medical Association* vol. 205, 1968, p. 855
11. Dobyns, B M *et al.*, *Journal of Clinical Endocrinology and Metabolism* vol. 38, 1974, p. 96
12. Hayek, A *et al.*, *New England Journal of Medicine* vol. 283, 1970, p. 949; Safa, A M *et al.*, *New England Journal of Medicine* vol. 292, 1975, p. 67; Freitas, J E *et al.*, *Journal of Nuclear Medicine* vol. 20, 1979, p. 847
13. Sheline, G E *et al.*, *Journal of Clinical Endocrinology and Metabolism* vol. 19, 1959, p. 127
14. Stoffer, S S and Hamburger, J I, *Journal of Nuclear Medicine* vol. 17, 1976, p. 146

15. Robertson, J S and Gorman, C A, *Journal of Nuclear Medicine* vol. 17, 1976, p. 826
16. Safa, A M *et al.*, *New England Journal of Medicine* vol. 292, 1975, p. 167
17. Einhorn, J *et al.*, *Acta Radiologica* vol. 11, 1972, p. 93
18. Maier, W P *et al.*, *American Journal of Surgery* vol. 147, 1984, p. 267
19. Kalk, W J, *Lancet* vol. 1, 1978, p. 291

## Chapter 6

1. *Transactions of the Clinical Society of London*, 'Report of a committee to investigate the subject of myxoedema', 1888, p. 21
2. Mackenzie, H W G, *British Medical Journal* vol. 2, 1892, p. 940
3. *See* Smith, Tom, *Heart Attack – Prevent and Survive* (3rd edn; Sheldon Press, 2000) for the details
4. Myerowitz, P D, *Journal of Thoracic and Cardiovascular Surgery* vol. 86, 1986, p. 57
5. J G Cooper and colleagues, *British Medical Journal* 2005, volume 330, page 1002

## Chapter 7

1. Roth, R N, *Emergency Medical Clinics of North America* vol. 7, 1989, p. 83

## Chapter 8

1. Parry, C H, *Collections from the unpublished papers of the late Caleb Hilliel Parry* (vol. 2; London: Underwoods, 1825)
2. Hoffman, W H *et al.*, *American Journal of Psychiatry* vol. 135, 1978, p. 484
3. Shaw, Dr C, 'Case of myxoedema with restless melancholia treated by injections of thyroid juice', *British Medical Journal* vol. 2, 1892, p. 451

## Chapter 10

1. Murray, G R, *British Medical Journal* vol. 2, 1891, p. 796

## Chapter 11

1. Thompson, N W *et al.*, *Current Problems in Surgery* vol. 15, 1978, p.1
2. Fogelfeld, L *et al.*, *New England Journal of Medicine* vol. 320, 1989, p. 835

# Index

Lightning Source UK Ltd.
Milton Keynes UK
UKOW051218241012

201121UK00001B/13/P